KELOID TREATMENT SECRETS

What Your Doctor Won't Tell You

MICHAEL H. TIRGAN, MD

ISBN-13: 978-1515366393
ISBN-10: 1515366391
LCCN: 2015913682

BISAC: Medical / Dermatology

Publisher: CreateSpace Independent Publishing Platform, North Charleston, SC, USA

Printed in the United States of America

Dedication

Dedicated to all those who suffer from keloid disorder.

About The Author

Michael H. Tirgan, M.D. is a board-certified medical oncologist.

He is also the only doctor in North America currently specializing in the research and treatment of keloid disorder.

Dr. Tirgan's practice is solely focused on the treatment of patients who have keloid disorder. In the years since he started his practice, he has treated all manner of keloids and helped more than 900 patients.

His practice focuses on non-surgical treatments and serves both adults and children.

In addition to his extensive clinical experience with keloid disorder, Dr. Tirgan has contributed to the effort to develop effective treatments by publishing peer-reviewed articles based on his research.

He is currently the leading expert on keloid disorder.

Table of Contents

Introduction

Imagine a disorder where the body's own healing process becomes a source of lifelong misery.

Imagine scar-like growths that spread from the ear to the face, or that expand to encompass and compromise the joints.

Imagine the growths becoming so severe that they rob you of your hearing as they invade your ears.

A girl goes to get her ears pierced. Rather than going through the normal healing process, her ears scar, swell with fibrous tissues and eventually end up deformed.

A simple act of decoration, a rite of passage even, initiates horrible suffering.

A child or adult bounces from general practitioner to dermatologist to plastic surgeon to get these growths treated. Surgery after surgery only leads to worsening growths and dashed hopes, after all that expense and pain.

The patient eventually gives up, their quality of life diminished and the growths expanding far beyond where they would have had they not been operated on in the first place.

These scenarios, and so many others that are equally painful, describe keloid disorder, and how it affects those who suffer from it.

Keloid disorder is classified as a cosmetic disorder. It is far more than that.

It has the power to destroy people's self-esteem. It has the power to lessen their chances in life, not because there is anything about keloid sufferers that makes them damaged or less capable than any other human being, but because of social prejudices. It happens because of the value that we, as human beings, attach to a person's physical appearance, whether we admit to doing so or not.

Within these pages I hope to give you some idea of what keloid disorder is and how it should and should not be treated. I will offer information on what types of research are needed to work toward tests for the disorder, treatments for sufferers and, perhaps, a cure.

I will also detail why there has been so little interest in this disorder.

I hope that, if you suffer from keloid disorder, this book will bring you at least that comfort that comes with an increased knowledge of what's going on with your body.

If you don't personally suffer from this disorder, than I hope it enlightens you as to the misery this disorder causes in so many people's lives.

There needs to be more awareness of this disorder, but the deck is stacked against those who suffer from it.

The emphasis on profit before patients in the medical community, institutional resistance and the simple fact that this disorder mainly affects a population that enjoys less access to healthcare than most others put keloid sufferers in a terrible position.

Where there should be knowledge, there is ignorance.

Where there should be research, there is inaction.

Where there should be treatments, there are procedures that often make the condition worse.

Worst of all, where there should be a voice, there is mostly silence.

I hope this book helps to change all of those things.

If you are a keloid sufferer, I also sincerely hope that you feel better informed and better equipped to deal with keloid disorder once you've finished it.

Michael H. Tirgan, M.D.

CHAPTER 1

Keloid Disorder Is More Complex Than Your Doctors Realize

In this chapter, you'll learn:

- What Keloid Disorder is and is not
- That the medical community lacks significantly in the tools required to treat keloid disorder
- That keloid disorder is an inherited condition
- That precautions should be taken for your children if you are a parent that suffers with this disorder

Keloid disorder is a disorder of the skin. It is notable for the sometimes large and often recurring tumors it causes in those affected.

It is also notable for being particularly difficult to treat.

In fact, not only is keloid disorder difficult to treat, but many of the treatments currently pursued by sufferers actually exacerbate the symptoms of the disorder.

Even the vocabulary used to discuss keloid disorder is, in many ways, inaccurate.

Keloid Disorder Is Not Scarring

If you suffer from keloid disorder, you may have had the characteristic skin tumors described as "scars" or "scarring."

This is inaccurate.

Keloids are the result of a genetic skin *disorder*, not normal scarring. The disorder, however, has a strong connection to the way the body heals, a process which doesn't function normally in persons who suffer from it.

When a person without keloid disorder receives some sort of trauma to the skin, such as an incision from surgery, and accidental laceration, a tattoo or a piercing, their body goes through a rather predictable healing cycle.

The skin fuses back together, some scar tissue forms and, through a very complex biological system, the body arrests the healing process once it's complete.

In a keloid disorder sufferer, the negative feedback loop that informs the body that it's time to stop the healing process doesn't function as it should.

This eventually creates collagen and/or glycoprotein deposits in the skin. That, in turn, manifests as the characteristic tumors.

The tumors may be large or small, in groups or dispersed across the skin. Some sufferers have only one, small affected area on their body. Others have extensive coverage, sometimes affecting twenty or thirty percent of their skin.

Some people will develop keloids after a seemingly insignificant trauma, such as an ear piercing. This is a common manifestation of the disorder, in fact, and often results in a mushroom-like growth that extends out beyond the edges of the ear, causing significant disfigurement, in some cases.

Other sufferers may endure a significant amount of skin trauma before the disorder manifests. This is commonly observed in patients who are middle aged or older and seek cosmetic surgery. Months after the surgery has healed, the symptoms of keloid disorder may appear for the first time in their lives.

An important thing to keep in mind about keloid disorder is that, even if the sufferer only manifests their first symptoms at middle age, they've had it for their entire life.

Keloid Disorder Is Genetic

For those few physicians and researchers who have invested their time, money and sweat into researching this disorder, its genetic origins do provide a way for them to at least make a risk assessment for patients, offsetting somewhat the lack of a sophisticated diagnostic tool.

If you have keloid disorder, your children are at a higher risk of having it. The same applies if your brother, sister, mother or father or other close relatives have suffered from it.

Keloid disorder is genetic; this much is understood. The frustrating lack of research or even interest in the disorder, discussed in later chapters, leaves a significant void in determining whether or not a person actually has the disorder, however, at least until it manifests.

Currently, there is no way to test for keloid disorder. There is no diagnostic tool that a physician can use to definitively determine whether or not you or a loved one might have it.

However, if it runs in your family, it's advantageous to assume that younger members of the family that may not have presented with a tumor yet do suffer from keloid disorder, and to take appropriate cautions. These would include:

- Not getting ears pierced
- Not getting tattoos
- Being cautious about any activities that may cause skin trauma
- Finding effective treatment as soon as symptoms do manifest

As you'll also find out in later chapters, that last recommendation is enormously difficult, for myriad reasons.

The point about being cautious is particularly relevant for younger people.

Keloid Disorder Tends to Manifest First in Adolescents

Most people first exhibit signs of keloid disorder between the ages of fifteen and sixteen. It may strike children as young as nine months old, however, or be present without manifesting until someone is around twenty-five years of age.

To add to the frustrating lack of medical knowledge of the disorder, there is currently very little to go on in terms of predicting when in a person's life keloid disorder will present.

Physicians that treat the disorder have to rely on very old medical reports, in some cases, and what scant new material has been produced in recent years.

Keloid Disorder Tends to Affect Certain Populations More than Others

African Americans have the highest rate of keloid disorder. People with darker complexions are more likely to develop it than those with lighter complexions, in general.

That's not to say that people with light skin are immune. People with very light skin, in fact, can suffer from this disorder, though the rates among lighter-skinned people are lower than they are among other populations.

People of Asian heritage suffer from keloid disorder at a higher percentage than other populations, as well.

It can affect anyone, however. No one is immune.

The Severity of Injuries Affects the Severity of the Tumors

Keloids will develop to a degree that's proportional to the cause.

For example, someone who develops a keloid tumor due to an ear piercing may develop the commonly seen mushroom-shaped mass in the area where they were pierced.

Someone who gets an open gallbladder surgery, however, may develop a much larger mass of tissue after the wound has healed.

This relationship between the level of trauma a patient experiences and the severity of the keloid they develop plays into how ineffective—and sometimes counterproductive—some treatments for keloid disorder tend to be, as you'll discover in coming chapters.

One of the worst scenarios that some of my patients face comes after healing from a cosmetic surgery. Not having suffered any major skin trauma in the past, they have the surgery done, unaware that they have keloid disorder.

After the surgery heals, the disorder manifests in the characteristic tumors in the areas where the patient endured incisions and other trauma from the surgery.

The end result for such individuals can be very severe and psychologically devastating.

As you'll learn in coming chapters, there are different types of keloids, as well, some of which are seen in some populations more than others.

Keloid Disorder Is More than Cosmetic

Insurance companies classify keloid disorder as a cosmetic disorder.

When someone has keloids over twenty to thirty percent of their body, when some of those keloids cause other issues, such as mobility problems with their joints, the disorder can hardly be called cosmetic any longer.

In fact, calling it such minimizes the harm it can do.

While there is a significant gap in scientific knowledge of this disorder, there are some studies that have been done into the impacts it has on people's lives. What those studies revealed is distressing.

A study entitled *Keloids: Assessment of effects and psychosocial-impacts on subjects in a black African population*, published in 2008 by the Department of Surgery, Lautech Teaching Hospital in Osogbo, Osun State, Nigeria, revealed much.

That study involved patients of the Plastic Surgery Clinic at the aforementioned teaching hospital. There were 131 patients involved in total, which included sixty-one males and seventy females. The majority of the patients had been living with a keloid lesion for at least a year.

The study found that:

- Twelve percent of the participants said that the keloid had impacted their work
- More than forty-eight percent said that they had been stigmatized due to their disorder
- Fifty-six percent said that they had lesions that were on noticeable parts of their body, while the remainder had them in inconspicuous locations
- More females felt stigmatized than did males
- 35.8 percent felt that their keloid had limited their social interactions

Nigeria is a nation where keloid disorder is endemic and where people are likely to be more familiar with the characteristic lesions.

In the US, we face the same problem that you'll see referenced again and again in this book when assessing the psycho-social impacts of keloid disorder: a lack of research.

What we do know is that people in the US have a hard time dealing with disfiguring conditions, both on the part of the affected and on the part of those around them.

In the 1970s, social scientists performed a study that examined how people deal with disfigurement in others.

Most people feel an urge to stare at disfigured individuals. This is understandable; disfigurement is anomalous in our everyday experiences. Fortunately, the social prohibition against staring inhibits most people from indulging that reflexive response.

Unfortunately, though the way such individuals act to

preserve the dignity of the affected is admirable, it results in avoidance. Avoidance, of course, results in the disfigured individual becoming isolated.

People with keloid disorder have to deal with a great many social difficulties. These include the aforementioned avoidance, but may also include other behaviors on the part of the people the sufferer interacts with that are equally distressing.

Some individuals may take a pitying attitude toward a keloid sufferer. Ask anyone with a disfiguring condition or a handicap how being pitied feels and you're likely to get a very negative response!

Some individuals, perhaps well meaning, may ask very personal questions or render advice to the affected individual. You'll learn about the frustration that keloid sufferers deal with further along in the book, but imagine how it feels, after having visited doctor after doctor, to have a complete stranger render unsolicited, and likely completely ignorant, advice.

In some cases, people who suffer with keloid disorder deal with much worse and, particularly in younger individuals, this may be very psychologically, and possibly physically, dangerous. Some people who look different are bullied because of it, and that can cause very real harm.

It's important to keep in mind that the bullying that keloid sufferers experience may not be physical. It may be emotional or it may be exhibited as simple avoidance by their peers. The sufferer may grow to feel remarkably isolated after a time.

Combine all of these things together and, if you have any kind of character, you'll only feel compassion.

Compassion is important and useful, but it's not a treatment option and, no matter how understanding one person is, it's likely that people's general ignorance of this disorder will cause them to react negatively to someone who has a significant amount of keloid coverage over a highly-conspicuous area of their body.

Put yourself in such an individual's shoes for a moment, if you don't suffer this disorder yourself, and you'll quickly realize how hard life could be.

Cosmetic condition, indeed.

There is, however, one important thing you should understand about keloid disorder before we move on, if only for your peace of mind.

Keloid Disorder Is Not Deadly

Nodules and other features that grow on the skin; odd colorations; pain, itching and other symptoms: keloid disorder can be frightening.

It also involves the uncontrolled production of tissue on the part of the body. These symptoms together sound an awful lot like a word no one ever wants their doctor to say to them: cancer.

Keloid disorder is not cancer. The difference between the two is simple enough: cancer can kill you; keloid disorder will not.

Keloid tumors are benign. That, in fact, is what makes it easy for insurance companies and the medical world at large to write off keloid disorder as a cosmetic problem, though it can be, and often is, much more than that.

It's important to remember that, simply because a condition doesn't threaten your life, it doesn't follow that it doesn't threaten your *quality* of life.

Keloid disorder can be devastating. If you or a family member suffer from it, you already know this. If you're a parent, it's probably crossed your mind more than once that your child might suffer from this disorder.

That may well be the case.

Know, however, that your life is not in danger from keloid disorder. While that might not help you with the social anxiety, body image issues and other hardships that come with this disorder, it should, at least, put your mind at ease about whether or not your life is at risk.

You may already know that because of having visited a medical professional for treatment.

In the next chapter, we'll go over the different types of keloids. They differ in more than appearance. To some degree, I have been able to successfully treat them for my patients, but there is still much that needs to be done in finding effective ways to help people who suffer with keloids.

Chapter 2

There Are Many Different Types of Keloids and Each Requires Different Treatments

In this chapter you'll learn:

- That keloids come in many different shapes
- That some types of keloids can cause accompanying physical problems
- That some keloids are known to cause pain
- That treatment options vary according to the type of keloid in question

Keloids, in addition to presenting in different levels of severity, can manifest in different shapes.

The causes of these different shapes are currently unknown. There are some characteristic symptoms that go along with each type, however.

Let's take a look at the shapes that keloids come in. The

shape of your keloid will likely, to some extent, dictate the best possible treatment for the tumor.

Flat Keloids

Flat keloids, just as the name implies, do not rise above the level of the skin to any meaningful degree. They tend to occur more often in people with lighter skin tones, including Asians, but they affect African Americans and other people with darker skin tones, as well.

Flat keloids can appear in a variety of different shapes. Some of them may have a butterfly shape to them; others might simply look like a disorganized mass with irregular borders.

Flat keloids are associated with other, accompanying symptoms that make them harder to endure for some patients.

Flat keloids should not be treated surgically. As is the case with most types of keloids, this course of treatment is likely to result in the formation of an even more pronounced keloid after the healing process has completed.

For these types of keloids, I generally recommend cryotherapy, along with chemotherapy, in some cases.

Steroid treatment is also an option for these types of keloids and the results are sometimes quite good. Unfortunately, there are instances where steroid treatment may actually result in flat keloids becoming worse.

Like other types of keloids, there are limited treatment options for flat keloids and, quite often, they simply go untreated. Also like other types of keloids, these can come in varying degrees of severity and can grow over time.

These keloids may be of the hyper-inflammatory type, which is discussed later in this chapter.

Nodular Keloids

Nodular keloids extend above the level of the skin. In some instances, they may actually have a stalk-like structure.

These types of keloids may appear somewhat like a large mole, but they are much different. They may appear singularly or in groups and can form in different sizes.

These types of keloids may grow to as large as two centimeters in size.

Linear Keloids

The name given to these types of keloids describes them well; they appear as lines on the body.

They may be raised above the skin somewhat and look very much like scars.

Treatment for these keloids employs the same range of options used to treat other types of keloids.

Guttate Keloid

These types of keloids have something of a teardrop shape to them, from which they take their name.

Guttate keloids may appear in groups, which can make them particularly damaging in the cosmetic sense. They are treated in the same manner as other types of keloids and, unfortunately, knowledge of their exact cause and treatment options are both as limited as they are with other types of keloids.

Guttate keloids can appear anywhere, but they tend to manifest most often on the arms and the trunk.

Superficially Spreading Keloids

These are among the most distressing types of keloids, and they can grow quite large over time. They also present among the most significant challenges to treatment.

These keloids can grow large enough to encompass a significant area of skin, causing body image issues and significant psychological distress.

It can get worse.

Should one of these keloids form near a joint and grow to a large enough size, it may actually impact mobility. Even when they do not, they are likely to impact how comfortable one feels taking off clothing for activities such as swimming and sports, which could have a negative impact on the sufferer's quality of life.

Treating superficially spreading keloids is very difficult. Chemotherapy drugs may be used to treat these tumors. In other cases, steroids are employed, particularly when chemotherapy drugs are not appropriate for the patient.

Someone suffering from significant keloids of this type likely faces a lot of personal and social difficulties as a result, and may experience physical problems, as well. The keloids are not, however, cancerous and are not a threat to the patient's life.

Massive Keloids

Massive keloids can grow to very large sizes, as the name indicates. They are notoriously hard to treat, though cryotherapy has proven to be one of the best possible options.

These keloids can be disfiguring. They may appear on the ears or on other parts of the body.

This type of keloid is exclusively seen in people of African American and African heritage. Those with darker skin tones are most affected by this particular manifestation of keloid disorder.

One of the very disturbing aspects of this type of keloid is that it can form without any apparent cause. While trauma to the skin is strongly associated with the formation of keloids, massive keloids can form at any time, with no apparent trauma that led to them presenting on the patient.

While there are no diagnostic tools to test for the risk of these types of keloids, there are some observed commonalities between patients that are useful to be aware of:

- A family history of keloid disorder
- Early onset of keloids
- The condition being exacerbated by chicken pox
- New keloids developing after minor skin injuries
- Rapid development of new keloids
- Hypertension at an early age

There are some treatments that are specifically contraindicated for this type of keloid, and that may make the condition worse. They include:

- Radiation therapy
- Surgery

Unfortunately, there are limited treatment options for this type of keloid, and there is much research that needs to be done. Ideally, a treatment option would be systemic, and would provide some level of control over the development of new keloids.

These keloids can become so extensive that they take up the majority of large areas of skin, including the back, chest and other parts of the body, and can seriously impact the sufferer's self-esteem and body image.

Hyper-Inflammatory Keloid

Keloids of this type tend to be of the flat variety. What differentiates them from other types of keloids is that they cause pain; sometimes significant amounts of it.

These keloids can be painful enough, in fact, to seriously impact the affected individual's quality of life. The pain may be accompanied by itching and other symptoms. They appear quite frequently on the chest, right around the mid-point.

The pain associated with these keloids can be distracting and is sometimes noticeable at all times.

I work with patients suffering this disorder in two ways.

- First, I try to control the amount of pain and discomfort they experience. Relieving the pain, in and of itself, can be of significant benefit to the patient.

- Second, I treat the keloid itself, oftentimes employing chemotherapy drugs.

Because of the pain associated with these types of keloids, sufferers tend to have tried everything possible to deal with them by the time they become my patient, including surgery.

In some cases, physicians may have completely given up on a patient by the time they come to see me. The pain, however, might have been going on for years, to the point where the patient can't even touch the affected area.

I have been able to significantly reduce the pain that these sufferers experience, allowing them to avoid hardships such as interrupted sleep and even difficulty wearing certain clothing.

Dealing with Frustration

There are many different types of keloids, as has been discussed, and there are significant differences in the level and type of hardship they cause in people's lives.

One thing that tends to remain consistent, however, is the patient trying a variety of different therapies, with results that either fail to provide relief or that actually end up making their condition worse.

As the only specialist in this field, I have been able to successfully treat some patients and to provide significant relief to others.

However, there is so precious little that is known about this disorder at present, and such a lack of interest in studying it further that, for the moment, keloid sufferers remain one of the most under-recognized and underserved of all groups seeking medical treatment.

As you've learned, this lack of options can have very negative consequences. Imagine living with constant pain and itching, having your face grow ever more disfigured, or having to go out in public with large masses growing from your ears.

This is not a cosmetic disorder. The fact that it is classified as such is just one more demonstration of the lack of care and simple compassion available to people who suffer from keloids.

While I have been able to achieve some degree of success where others have not, it remains the case that those with keloid disorder often suffer mightily and, as you'll learn, finding ways to offer them relief, or to even research options for doing so, is a struggle in and of itself.

In the next chapter, we're going to discuss why visiting a dermatologist or surgeon, the two types of practitioners that keloid sufferers are likely to seek out, may be the wrong course of action.

Either choice is logical, so don't feel like you've made a mistake of some sort if you have sought relief from your condition from one of the aforementioned medical professionals.

Like you, they probably know little about keloid disorder. They may have done the best they could for you and had only the most admirable of intentions, but the treatment options they pursued may have made things worse.

You may already be aware of that, in fact.

CHAPTER 3

The Most Commonly-Sought Treatments Can Make Keloid Disorder Worse

n this chapter, you'll learn that:

- Some of the treatments commonly ordered for keloid disorder actually worsen the tumors
- Some of the treatments are very dangerous
- The usual pathway to treatment taken by sufferers is generally ineffective
- Surgery is your worst enemy in treating keloid disorder

When something is wrong with your skin, you likely seek out a dermatologist right away. When you want something removed from your body, you likely seek out a surgeon.

You're generally correct to do so, in most cases.

But not with Keloid disorder.

As you'll discover in this chapter, Keloid disorder is quite often made worse by the treatments most people pursue.

It's important to keep in mind as you're reading this that none of it is intended to call into question the qualifications or intentions of any physician you've frequented. They meant the best; they tried their best.

The problem is that there is so little knowledge of Keloid disorder in the medical community that the treatments ordered are sometimes the worst possible courses of action. The outcomes, sadly, are predictably negative, in many cases.

The Usual Path Keloid Sufferers Take

In instances where children manifest keloid disorder and their parents are also sufferers, the child may be at something of an advantage compared to many others. Their parents may have tried some treatments, had poor outcomes and might avoid trying them for their children.

In other cases, however, those children's parents will usually follow a rather predictable course of action. Adults that develop keloid disorder later in life will usually follow this same pattern.

The patient will usually see a general practitioner first. The general practitioner, not being an expert in skin conditions but being clearly presented with one, will refer the child—or adult, if that's who is suffering—to a dermatologist.

The dermatologist will typically use steroid injections for most patients. This can have some benefits but, as you'll learn, there are some potentially negative consequences, as well.

The steroid treatments may become rather intensive after a time. If a little doesn't do it, a lot more of the same treatment might be applied to the condition.

This is not at all without consequences. In any case where the amount of medication a patient receives is increased, the side effects of that medication increase, as well.

With steroid treatments, the side effects include:

- Skin discoloration
- Loss of skin tissue
- Cushing's syndrome

The last of those side effects, Cushing's syndrome, can be disfiguring. It can cause puffiness and redness in the face, the development of fatty deposits on the body—commonly between the shoulders—and stretch marks.

Steroid injections can also be very painful, which causes some patients to abandon the therapy soon after beginning it.

Only about ten to fifteen percent of patients who opt to go through steroid injection see any kind of positive outcome. Some studies have shown that more than fifteen percent of patients will actually experience a worsening of the condition.

Steroids are heavily marketed to dermatologists. They are, in many cases, the go-to treatments for various skin conditions. Quite often, they are very effective and provide significant relief to people suffering a variety of different problems with their skin.

Where keloid disorder is concerned, however, steroid treatments have marginal results, at best, and the side effects of treatment may make it unendurable.

Add to this that there is no established dosage for treating keloid disorder with steroids and you have a situation where more is likely to be called for, with ever-worsening results, if there are any results at all.

Plastic Surgery

The surgeon's knife, even in this era of very advanced medical technology, is one of the most powerful healing tools available. Surgery is a suitable treatment for a wide variety of different conditions, ranging from the worst cancers to elective cosmetic procedures.

Where keloid disorder is concerned, however, surgery is likely to make things much worse.

It is not unusual or unwise that people seek out surgeons to get rid of keloids; it is an action that is simply uninformed.

When something presents itself on your body—a mole, a skin tag, even a wrinkle—the most natural and effective course of action is quite often to have a skilled surgeon treat it.

In the case of keloid disorder, however, it's important to keep the cause of the disorder in mind when assessing the suitability of surgery as a treatment option.

Keloid disorder is caused by trauma to the skin, and surgery is a major trauma.

In fact, in many cases, the keloid will not only make a return after being surgically removed, but will actually be worse when it comes back.

The trauma from the surgical incision will likely be much more severe than the trauma that caused the keloid to appear and, therefore, will result in a much larger keloid. This cycle could go on endlessly, of course.

There is one specific type of keloid where surgery may be an option. When keloids develop that depend or extend from the ear, what we call a pedunculated keloid that does not involve full thickness of any part of the ear, and in a patient who has no other keloids, removing them surgically may result in a positive outcome for the patient.

In all other cases, however, surgery is not an advisable treatment for keloid disorder. It sometimes seems to be the most logical course of action, but it's far more likely to exacerbate the keloid that was removed.

Months after the surgery, when everything seems to be healing correctly, the keloid will very likely come back, and with a vengeance.

Unless you have a pedunculated keloid on your ear, make no mistake: surgery is your worst enemy.

Unfortunately, assessing the precise amount of risk of recurrence or potential worsening of keloids following surgical removal is really an impossible task for physicians. There is simply too little research to go on.

What is known, however, is that some types of keloids are almost certain to reappear following a surgical excision. The addition of accompanying treatments may lessen these odds, at least on some areas of the body but, again, those treatments might come at significant risk to the patient.

Sometimes, in fact, they may involve deadly risks.

Radiation Therapy

I'll start off this section with a simple piece of advice: Don't do this.

Radiation therapy is dangerous. In some cases, it's a cancer patient's best hope of surviving and, in treating cancers, it can offer remarkable results.

Those situations are life-and-death in nature. Using this modality as an option for keloid treatment may result in a life-or-death situation that never had to occur.

There was a time when radiation therapy was used to treat certain skin conditions such as acne or fungal infections of the scalp. Over the decades, this has been abandoned. There is one simple reason for this.

Radiation therapy increases your risk of cancer.

Moreover, the cancers that result from radiation therapy tend to be very difficult to treat.

Radiation therapy may be employed following a surgical treatment for keloid disorder. It may or may not help. The harm it may do can include severe damage to the organs and, of course, the development of potentially deadly cancers.

I highly recommend that you do not consent to radiation treatments for keloid disorder. It is not likely to result in an improvement of your keloid and it may do the worst possible kind of damage to your body.

If you are among the people who have already received radiation treatments for keloids, I encourage you to seek out the Keloid Radiation Registry. This is a resource that's designed to provide concrete data on the safety of radiation treatments for keloids, and whether it has any real benefit.

Cryoshape

Cryoshape is sometimes recommended as a treatment for keloids, but it is not one I endorse, for several different reasons.

Cryoshape is a very invasive form of cryotherapy. There is no hard evidence indicating that this procedure is any more effective than regular cryotherapy, which is far less invasive.

There is also a lack of control on the part of the operator. This procedure involves sticking a very large needle through the keloid and freezing the tissue with liquid nitrogen. During this process, the person operating the device has no way of knowing how far the freezing has extended—possibly into healthy tissue—and no way of controlling the depth of the freezing, even if they did.

This, combined with the heightened risk of infection and side effects, which include oozing and other unpleasant results, make it inappropriate for keloid therapy. I do not recommend that patients pursue this option.

On top of its other drawbacks, this procedure is another that introduces even more trauma to the affected area in the form of the cryoshape device itself being inserted, as well as the injections used to numb the area prior to the procedure being administered.

Knowledge and Specialists Are Both Lacking

Part of the issue with ineffective treatments so often being ordered stems from there being very little hard research done into Keloid disorder.

Another significant barrier to patients getting effective treatment is the lack of specialists in this area. In fact, I am currently the only physician specializing in this particular disorder.

While any physician trying to treat you is certainly doing their level best to ensure the most positive possible outcome, the lack of knowledge in the medical community and, as you'll learn, the lack of interest in researching this disorder with the diligence it merits, both result in a situation where the cures ordered often actually worsen the disease, and lower the quality of life of the patients seeking treatment.

effective treatment is the lack of specialists in this area. In fact, I am currently the only physician specializing in this particular disorder.

While any physician trying to treat you is certainly doing

their level best to ensure the most positive possible outcome, the lack of knowledge in the medical community and, as you'll learn, the lack of interest in researching this disorder with the diligence it merits, both result in a situation where the cures ordered often actually worsen the disease, and lower the quality of life of the patients seeking treatment.

Chapter 4

Keloid Disorder Should Not Influence Your Pursuit of Necessary Medical Procedures

In this chapter, you'll learn:

- That keloid disorder makes some medical decisions very difficult

- That some necessary treatments may make your condition worse

- That you should not forego necessary treatments due to the fear of developing new keloids

You've already learned a lot about keloid disorder. You've also learned that many of the recommended treatments are actually detrimental to addressing the disorder.

In this chapter, we're going to discuss one of the most important things you should understand if you or someone close to you suffers from this disorder.

Some Exacerbating Procedures Are Still Necessary

You may find yourself in a situation where a surgeon calls for a surgery that is absolutely necessary for your health. It might be an appendectomy, the removal of a cancerous mole, a caesarian section or another treatment that will inevitably involve trauma to the skin.

These treatments, of course, will mean that a keloid will almost certainly form in the area where the incision is made.

Given the severe trauma involved in a surgical incision and the way that keloids form in proportion to the amount of trauma received, it's also almost inevitable that the keloid will be rather severe.

You should still have the procedure done.

Necessary Procedures and Body Image

Do not think yourself vain if you hesitate to have what might be a necessary procedure out of fear of developing a severe keloid.

Fear of being disfigured is natural. As I've already pointed out, insurance companies unfairly classify keloid disorder as a cosmetic condition. As I've also pointed out, when you have keloids covering twenty or thirty percent of your body, or when they're in areas that are normally visible, the disorder is much more than cosmetic.

- It is life-changing.
- It affects your self-esteem.
- It affects how people look at you.

These are not insignificant points, and they're worth exploring.

As a keloid sufferer, you have a valid concern and, unfortunately, the ways in which surgeons and other medical professionals may calm fears of disfigurement in other patients might not apply to you.

Fixing the Damage

For the sake of example, let's use someone who isn't like you or anyone who suffers from keloid disorder. Let's use someone whose condition is the result of a voluntary behavior.

Imagine someone who has spent their lifetime chewing tobacco and, predictably enough, ends up with oral cancer. That individual may require radical surgery, including the removal of a great deal of tissue.

The fact that they, for the most part, brought this upon themselves should not dampen our compassion for such an individual. We all make bad decisions, after all, and if addictions weren't dangerously hard to abandon, they wouldn't merit the name "addiction," which comes from a Latin term which means "surrender."

Facing a surgery that would almost certainly involve significant disfigurement to their face, the patient's healthcare providers would likely comfort the patient by letting them know about the advanced nature of reconstructive surgery. Scarring can be reduced. Destroyed tissues can be rebuilt. Oral surgeons can replace lost teeth and fix other issues.

It's a painful remedy, of course, but one that is likely to result in at least some comfort for the patient.

For a keloid sufferer, however, the situation is much different.

As I've pointed out, there is precious little understanding of this disorder in the medical community. Where there is understanding, there is still a gaping void in terms of diagnostic and therapeutic tools that can treat the condition.

For keloid disorder sufferers, that reconstructive surgery is likely to result in more keloids. Each procedure, in fact, may make the keloid disorder more severe.

So, what is a keloid disorder sufferer to do?

If it's necessary to preserve your health and, certainly, if a procedure is required to preserve your very life, then you must get it.

Hard Choices

Some moles have to be removed, even if the removal is going to result in a keloid.

Some births are likely to be so dangerous to the mother, child or both that a caesarian section must be performed.

Do not forgo a necessary medical procedure because of fear of developing more keloids. It is true that, excepting myself, there is no one practicing that specializes in this disorder. There are few routes available to you if you develop new or worse keloids that need treatment. Nonetheless, to forgo a procedure that may save your life to avoid worsening one that poses no threat to your life at all makes no sense.

In coming chapters, we will discuss the frustrating situation that I and the few other parties interested in learning more about diagnosing and treating keloid disorder face.

You'll also learn that there is hope for treating this disorder.

As it stands, surgical trauma is very likely to worsen your condition, however. Again, as traumatic as that may be, please do not let the very real psychological hardships that keloid disorder oftentimes entails dissuade you from pursuing a necessary course of treatment.

It's a hard choice to make, but it's certainly better to live with a disorder than it is to perish from a disease that might be treatable, even if the treatment is more than likely going to worsen your keloid disorder.

This is a short chapter, but this point is important enough that it merits its own section in this book. I sincerely hope you will take it to heart and never pass up a necessary treatment due to worries about your keloid disorder and, if you have a loved one who is thinking of doing so, that you will do everything in your power to encourage them to make the right choice.

As was said in the first chapter, however, elective procedures—even something as minor as ear piercing—can result in the formation of keloids. If you have a family member with this disorder or know that you have it yourself, do not get a cosmetic procedure done, do not get your ears pierced, a tattoo, a brand or any other decoration that will cause trauma to the skin.

If you do, you are very likely to develop a keloid. If you have a particularly severe case of keloid disorder, even a minor injury can result in the formation of a keloid, which may grow over time to become significant enough to cause disfigurement and all the other hardships that go along with it.

The same applies to the treatments I've already mentioned

that are known to make keloid disorder worse. To treat keloid disorder, do not get surgery; do not get cryoshape; do not get radiation.

Up until now, we've focused on the difficult issues that go along with keloid disorder. While the next chapter will likely give you a bit of hope, there is still much that needs to be done about this disorder and very few people and institutions willing to take it on.

It's remarkable to me that a disorder that may impact whether or not someone makes the correct decision in a life-or-death situation is still regarded as cosmetic.

Hopefully, this next chapter will shed a little light for you, because I and some other researchers are working toward a viable medical treatment for keloid disorder, but it's a long and hard road ahead.

CHAPTER 5

Medical Professionals Are Seeking New Treatments

I n this chapter, you'll learn:

- That keloid research is woefully underfunded
- That the level of research it merits is very expensive
- That I am actually the *only* physician specializing in keloid treatment
- That there is some hope, despite all of this

If you have keloid disorder, you've probably spent at least some time browsing the Internet for information on the disorder, and possible treatment options.

You've probably been disappointed in the results of your research, as well. There's good reason to be and I, myself, have experienced similar disappointment.

While there is some interest in keloid disorder among the medical community, you'll find that it's far less than one might expect.

Here are some things to consider, which are revealing in regards to why your own research efforts have likely yielded less than satisfactory, and certainly far from useful, results.

There Is Little Funding

In 2011, I started the Keloid Research Foundation (KRF). The KRF exists to foster research into keloid disorder. It also strives to advocate for those affected with the disorder and to provide educational resources for patients, their families and the public at large.

Unfortunately, it's been a very difficult enterprise studying this disorder in a comprehensive, scientific way. As I mentioned earlier, physicians seeking to treat the disorder sometimes have to rely on very old research and, where new research is concerned, there is very little to go on.

Many of these problems, as is the case with so many things, comes down to money. After four years, the KRF has approximately $2,000 in a bank account; obviously, not an amount that can be used to perform advanced research into the disorder.

Nonetheless, the vision of the KRF remains, and, provided more interest can be garnered from the medical community and the institutions that serve it, there is hope for a treatment for this disorder that is more effective than those presently available.

What Research Would Entail

We'll go further into what's involved with research in Chapter 8, but this should serve as an introduction.

If you follow cancer research, you're likely aware that

genetic research is a significant part of it. By studying the normal human genome, researchers are able to determine where the genes involved in cancer are located, how they differ in terms of being activated or suppressed and to gather other useful data.

That data can be, and has already been, used to develop effective treatments.

The KRF hopes to do the same with keloid disorder.

As you've already learned, keloid disorder is a genetic condition. It follows, therefore, that advanced study into the genetic characteristics of the disorder could lead to the development of drug therapies or other therapies that could reduce, or even cure, keloid disorder.

For the many people who suffer from this disorder, such a treatment would open up an entirely new world to them; a world where the psychological and physical suffering associated with the disorder could be reduced, or even eliminated.

The KRF believes that, by applying the most advanced genetic research techniques to keloid disorder, the medical community would be able to develop powerful new tools that could change the lives of millions of keloid sufferers forever.

Imagine not fearing that you or a loved one would develop disfiguring, painful keloids from even minor skin trauma. We can imagine such a world, to be certain, and the KRF means to make it a reality.

There Are Precedents

Consider, for a moment, what can happen when people come together to work toward a cure or treatment for a disorder or a disease. There are many such examples, and quite a few of them involve conditions that have far less impact on a sufferer's life than does keloid disorder.

Acne provides a good example. According to a study, *Epidemiology of acne vulgaris*, by K Bhate and HC Williams, the costs of treating acne exceed $3 billion per year in the United States alone.

In the quest to treat acne, which can cause significant harm in people's lives, make no mistake about that, antibiotics, anti-inflammatory drugs and other medical tools are employed.

As the study reveals, treating common acne is a multi-billion dollar industry. There are good reasons for that.

- Acne is disfiguring
- Acne can cause significant social anxiety
- Acne tends to strike people when they're at a vulnerable age, psychologically speaking
- Severe cases of acne can even lead to suicidal ideation

I challenge you: pick one of the above items that is also not true of keloid disorder.

Yet, the KRF struggles to get funding to conduct useful scientific research into the causes and possible treatments of keloid disorder.

A multi-billion dollar industry, versus $2,000 in a bank account.

But, we are determined.

In Some Ways, Keloid Disorder Is Worse

Continuing the comparison with acne, consider what was suggested in a previous chapter; that one should never forego a necessary medical treatment for fear of developing a keloid as a result.

When one considers that acne is not worsened by the same causes as keloid disorder, and that a surgery is not at all likely to result in worsening acne symptoms, it becomes clear that keloid disorder sufferers oftentimes face a more challenging decision than acne sufferers.

Yet, again, we have a multi-billion dollar industry and an incredibly useful body of research dedicated to treating acne, versus almost nothing to address keloid disorder.

The Complexities of Studies

We'll go into this topic to a far greater depth in Chapter 8, but here are some basics regarding the complexity of medical research.

Conducting medical studies is no small enterprise. It takes time, money, talent and many patients willing to undergo the study to arrive at useful results.

Those results can be powerful. In some cases, cancer sufferers, with their backs against a wall, will be offered participation in experimental treatments as an option. There are instances where those experimental treatments work for them, adding extra years to their life and an end to their awful suffering.

The KRF intends to do the same for keloid sufferers. More specifically, clinical trials are part of the agenda of the KRF.

Clinical research is a major undertaking. It requires patients, first and foremost, who can lend biological samples and other resources to the study and, sometimes, who are willing to participate in experimental treatments.

One route the KRF was interested in pursuing was the

use of certain drugs used to treat cancer for the treatment of keloid disorder. The FDA, however, disagreed with this approach, and the study could not be conducted.

We'll discuss this obstacle to research, and the many others, in coming chapters, but know that there are institutional barriers to research that sometimes make even applying known treatments for one condition to other conditions very difficult, indeed.

My background is in oncology, as was stated. There are similarities between keloid disorder and cancer that make exploring cancer treatments as options for keloid sufferers a natural pathway. This route, however, is not as accepted as I believe it should be among the medical community, but consider how the two diseases might be studied in similar ways.

In cancer research, biopsies of the cancerous tissues are widely-used and very effective tools. The same would logically apply to keloid disorder, which is, like cancer, a genetic condition that involves abnormal cell behavior.

Like cancer research, keloid research would logically involve a great degree of study into the genetics of the disorder. If you want an idea of why this is so meaningful as a methodology of research, consider what it could yield.

If you're a keloid sufferer, imagine being able to take your child to my office and have a test done.

Imagine being given a definitive answer to a question that's likely occupied more than enough of your time: Does your child have keloid disorder?

Further, imagine how this would impact your child's life. It would mean that the simple rites of passage that children go through as they reach adolescence and adulthood could be assessed as to their safety. You would know, for instance, if your child could safely get their ears pierced without having to take a risk and let them do it, with potentially devastating results.

It would mean that they could plan their medical treatments based on having or not having keloid disorder.

Moreover, it would mean that, if they did require medical treatments that involved skin trauma, there might actually be a treatment that could help them by reducing or completely eliminating the risk of developing keloids.

Right now, the treatments for keloids, even though I've enjoyed more success than other doctors in this regard, are lacking in several ways.

Currently, I and any other physicians seeking to offer a patient effective treatment are constrained to treating the affected area. All that is available to the medical community are treatments that depend upon a keloid being present, and us, as physicians, finding an effective way to eliminate, or at least reduce, the effects of the disorder.

The KRF envisions a world where drug therapies may prevent the disorder from manifesting in the first place and, if they do manifest, where the same or other drug therapies might safely eliminate keloids altogether.

It is a realistic vision. It is very much a vision that I wish more medical professionals and institutions shared in, but you're going to learn that there are significant barriers to making it a reality.

Most of those barriers are unnecessary. All of them are harmful, to greater or lesser degrees, to the sufferers of keloid disorder.

The KRF seeks to tear them down altogether.

In this next chapter, you'll learn about some of the treatment options I've used and what you might expect should you become a patient of mine.

CHAPTER 6

I Have Enjoyed Some Success

n this chapter, you'll learn:

- That I have had some success providing relief to patients
- That some of the treatments I've used are actually less invasive/radical than less-effective, but common, treatments
- That there are some cases of keloid disorder that cannot be treated at present

I have a busy practice providing care to people who suffer from keloid disorder. Some—many, actually—of the patients I've seen share similar histories and, before visiting me, they'd given up on treating their keloids altogether.

Let's start out by discussing some of the situations that I've commonly dealt with. They might be similar to your own and, if you've felt as if you were before, know that you are *not* alone.

Many Have Tried Other Treatments

Doctors can be clever, creative and quite innovative in their practice.

They can also be stubborn.

I have had people I know, people who trust me, get treatments for keloids that I knew would not work, even after I'd told them as much.

I cannot imagine how it must feel for patients when their doctors recommend a treatment that the patient knows will not or, worse, already has not, worked.

It's incredibly uncomfortable to contradict your doctor. After all, they put many years and a great deal of sweat into earning the right to wear that white coat, and it conveys authority for a reason.

It does not, however, mean that the person wearing it is always right.

When doctors are wrong about keloid treatments, the results are oftentimes disastrous, and I have seen this over and over again in my own practice.

In some cases, I'll get patients that have had surgeries on a primary keloid, which—predictably—resulted in a secondary keloid that was much worse.

These keloids can spread in disturbing and disfiguring ways. What started out as a small keloid on the ear may, after surgical removal, turn into a massive keloid that spreads across the entire ear or even onto the face. It may spread far below the surface of the skin.

Sometimes, the keloids may spread into the ear canal, robbing the patient of their hearing.

I see this far too often, and it gets worse.

Those patients that receive a failed surgery will often be recommended yet another. The next surgery, of course, will do nothing but cause the keloid to come back, and it will be worse.

Those secondary keloids will spread faster and farther than the primaries that were removed. They will sometimes be completely untreatable.

This is doubly tragic when you consider that, had the first keloid been given a treatment that was more appropriate, the secondary may have never formed.

Some of the patients, having endured suffering from both their keloid and surgeries, will simply give up. They'll let the keloid grow and grow, and it will grow fast.

What was a minor disfigurement will become a major source of mental misery. It will mean lost jobs, social ostracism and constant embarrassment.

It will mean stares, laughter from the less compassionate members of society and insecurity in the extreme.

Some of these patients may have given up, but I have not.

I have enjoyed some success in treating keloids, including severe examples. Sadly, there are some cases that I cannot treat.

Among the most significant things that differentiate me from so many of the other medical providers that my patients have visited in the past is that, if I'm presented with a case of keloid disorder that I cannot treat, I will not try.

That being said, there may be options for you if you haven't had any luck with other providers. This is my specialty and, for both the sake of giving information and, perhaps, as a way of giving you some hope, I wish to share with you the following.

Cryotherapy Can Work

We discussed cryotherapy previously, but let's go a bit further with the discussion, as it's one of the more effective ways to deal with certain types of keloids.

Cryotherapy works by destroying tissue. It's employed for a wide range of conditions, from warts to skin tags and beyond.

I typically utilize a specific method of cryotherapy that's likely a bit different than what you may have been recommended, but that has proven effective.

You may, for instance, have been recommended cryoshape, which was discussed earlier and which I strongly recommend against.

I apply cryotherapy to the keloid using a cotton swab. I do not spray the liquid nitrogen on and, as was said, I do not use cryoshape.

My choice of this method is backed up by research. In a study entitled *Cryotherapy in the treatment of keloids* conducted in 2006, there is evidence of the efficacy of this method.

That study, which involved 135 patients who had 166 keloids between them, tracked the results of cryosurgical treatments conducted between 1990 and 2004.

Of the 166 keloid masses treated, more than seventy-nine percent of them responded very well to the cryosurgery. They exhibited a reduction in mass in excess of eighty percent after the application of three treatments.

More than fourteen percent of the treated lesions showed a good response. Only six percent of cases involved responses that were less than satisfactory.

Those are all encouraging numbers, but there is one more statistic from this study that is even more striking.

No recurrences of the keloids were documented during the twelve to seventy-two month follow up period for participants.

The conclusion of that study:

> "*To date, cryotherapy appears to be the most effective, safe, economic, and easy-to-perform monotherapy to treat keloid lesions and hypertrophic scars.*" (Rusciani L 2006)

Cryotherapy is, in most cases, a patient's single best option toward getting relief from their condition, which is why I employ it.

If more doctors did the same, there would be less suffering from this disorder, to be certain.

Before you start searching the Internet, let me explain the type of cryotherapy I'm speaking about.

I'm not referencing the currently popular version wherein people go into spa-like settings to immerse themselves in chambers where they're exposed to sub-zero temperatures.

The cryotherapy I use is local. In fact, it's very precise. It targets the affected tissue alone. Unlike cryoshape, applying the liquid nitrogen with a cotton swab allows me very exact control over what tissue is affected.

Cryotherapy of this type has several benefits:

- It is targeted
- It has very minimal side effects
- Recovery is not particularly uncomfortable
- It is an established, trusted method of treatment

After the treatment, the tissue that has been subjected to cryosurgery will usually blacken. It may blister or ooze a bit.

The area is treated in the same way that one would treat an open wound, being covered with gauze and a loose dressing.

For most patients, it doesn't take long to heal.

The dead tissue sloughs off after the process has completed.

In some cases, there may be minor scarring or an altering of the pigmentation of the skin where the lesion was removed.

Other than that, the side effects are very minimal.

Cryotherapy is a safe and effective way to get rid of some keloids. For people who have a primary keloid they may have considered having surgically removed, receiving this treatment may well be the metaphorical equivalent of dodging a bullet.

Rather than going through a painful surgery, only to have a secondary keloid develop—likely much worse than the primary—the patient is left with their healthy tissue intact and without the fear that they're going to develop a more disfiguring lesion.

Steroid Therapy

This go-to treatment of dermatologists does have some value in treating keloids. It is not, however, as effective as cryotherapy, but may offer benefits in some cases.

I will employ this treatment where it may have benefit to the patient, but it is not a first-line therapy.

The side effects, as discussed on the chapter detailing ineffective treatments, can become severe if the amount of steroid used is excessive.

Of course, there is no established dosage for the steroid treatment of keloids.

Many patients come to me having already gone through

quite a few steroid treatments already. There are some keloids that are highly resistant to steroids and for which this course of action may be wholly ineffective.

There are some keloids, however, that do respond well to this treatment and, if it offers some benefit, it can be a good option.

Chemotherapy

Before you get too frightened, realize that this is not the same intense type of chemotherapy treatment that a serious cancer would require.

The drugs used, however, are sometimes the same ones used in treating some of the most dangerous of cancers.

Bleomycin is often employed as a treatment for testicular cancer and for Hodgkin's disease. This drug has been used with some success for keloid disorder.

Dr. Espana has a published paper on this course of treatment, which involved thirteen patients. Those patients did receive some relief from their keloids, with six of them having their keloids flatten.

Again, there is a strong connection between how keloids and cancers behave, so this treatment makes perfect sense.

His method of injecting the drugs utilized tattooing, and the drug is applied to the affected site, as opposed to being given intravenously or otherwise.

In a later chapter, you'll learn about how I tried to persuade the FDA to pursue using another anti-cancer drug for keloid treatment, and how frustrating it can be when a new idea is shot down by an institution simply because it deviates from the norm.

This particular cancer drug, Bleomycin, is already used

to treat conditions other than cancer. It's even used to treat some types of warts that are resistant to other treatments. It doesn't seem to have any systemic effects on the patients when applied using the tattooing method and when given in the low doses required for keloid treatment.

ScarFormula

ScarFormula is the brand name for a topically-applied cream that contains Panax ginseng. Unlike many other herbal remedies, ginseng has plenty of scientific studies to back up its efficacy in some situations and some of my patients have had good results from it.

This formula is used for the prevention of scars and the formation of keloids. It's designed to help in wound healing, as well.

In some patients, small keloids that may have developed into much larger problems were successfully regressed with this formula after long-term use.

This treatment may be used as an adjunct to other treatments. It's applied twice each day to all affected areas of the skin. I practice scientific medicine and, because of that, if results don't present themselves, the treatment may be discontinued.

ScarFormula may be used after cryotherapy, as well, to reduce the appearance of scars.

In the next chapter, we're going to explore one of the most significant reasons that the treatment options for keloid disorder are so limited.

The limitations, sadly, mostly stem from factors having nothing to do with the capabilities of modern research methods and the medicine that research can produce.

The limitations, in my opinion, should not exist.

CHAPTER 7

Socioeconomic Factors Play into the Lack of Treatments

n this chapter, you'll learn:

- That the quality of care that patients receive can be influenced by socioeconomic factors
- That conditions that affect mostly minority populations oftentimes go unaddressed
- That there is objective evidence supporting both of the above statements

Healthcare in the US is not received equally, or at the same degree of quality, across all races and socioeconomic classes.

This sad fact plays into the difficulty inherent in developing treatments and, potentially, cures for keloid disorder.

As you learned in previous chapters, keloid disorder tends

to disproportionately affect people of African American heritage and those with darker skin tones.

As you're going to learn, the way that this aspect of the disorder plays into securing money, time and support for research is not unusual and, unfortunately, a similar pattern has been observed again and again over the years.

African Americans and Healthcare in the US

African Americans are the second largest minority group in the United States, comprising 13.2 percent of the total population, according to 2014 US Census Bureau figures.

They are also twice as likely to live in poverty as are Asian Americans and Whites, according to a study by the Commonwealth Fund.

According to the same study, there are some rather distressing statistics related to how African Americans in the US interact with the healthcare system, their overall health, and the satisfaction they generally have with the quality of the care that they receive.

Statistics in a study entitled *Racial and Ethnic Disparities in U.S. Healthcare: A Chartbook*, reveal that forty-eight percent of African Americans between the ages of eighteen to sixty-four suffer from some sort of a chronic condition or disability.

This is in comparison to forty percent of whites, twenty-five percent of Asians and thirty-nine percent of the overall population.

The increased suffering continues as incomes go up. African Americans who earn more than the Federal Poverty

Level still suffer chronic conditions at higher rates than other racial groups in the US.

When one takes a look at similar statistics that concern access to healthcare, much the same is observed.

The study found that primary care physicians who have principally African American clients were more likely to report that they could not provide high-quality care to their patients.

African Americans, along with Hispanics, are also more likely to visit emergency rooms for conditions that could have, and likely should have, been handled by a primary care doctor.

They are also anywhere from two to four times more likely to be hospitalized for conditions that were preventable than are white Americans.

This all paints a picture wherein African Americans do not receive the same level of care from providers as do white Americans.

It follows, then, that a condition which strikes primarily those of African American heritage would not receive as much interest from the medical community as would one that either affected a typically more affluent group of patients or, at least, one that affected all racial groups more or less equally.

As is the case with the aforementioned billion-dollar medical industry dedicated to relieving acne.

All it takes is a brief Internet search to determine that there are many people out there suffering from keloid disorder, some of them significantly.

Given the statistics cited, it should come as no surprise that the largely African-American sufferers of this chronic condition receive little help from the medical community, and that there is not much in the way of research and development into new treatments and cures.

Suffering with Little Access to Help

The site ExperienceProject.com has a page where keloid disorder sufferers chat.

On that page, you'll hear familiar stories of the misery that goes along with this condition. The sufferers speak of not being able to find effective treatments. Many of them state the familiar complaint of having "tried everything," to no avail, of course.

Disclaimer: I'm mentioned on this site, quite favorably.

You'll also hear stories that should be familiar to you, now that you've read the previous chapters.

Patients go to get treatments and either have very unimpressive outcomes or, in some cases, their condition actually worsens.

While the posters on this site don't generally give their background information, given the typical sufferers of this condition, it's more than likely that most of them are African American or have dark-colored skin, particularly if they suffer from massive keloids.

Overall, they're not enjoying a positive experience with their healthcare providers.

Again, I'm not seeking to disparage any medical professional. It's quite simply that the treatments that are reflexively ordered for this condition do more harm than good.

- Plastic surgeons will want to perform surgeries.
- Dermatologists will want to inject steroids.

Neither is likely to be particularly effective and, more than likely, either will cause harm.

Left with inadequate treatment from their doctors, these keloid sufferers end up posting on the Internet.

Some of them receive understanding. Some of them receive advice that may or may not be constructive. Many are likely to resort to quack cures of one variety or another, or legitimate medical cures that, in the case of a keloid sufferer, simply are not going to work.

As a word of advice, "natural cures" can do real harm and the sites that advocate them are not typically run by anyone with real medical training or knowledge.

Thus, we're left with a situation where many of the people who suffer from keloid disorder simply have no obvious good option.

They can visit doctors with no treatments or answers, or go on the Internet to commiserate with other sufferers, but they are shut out from effective treatments.

As I've said, I'm the only physician currently specializing in keloid disorder. However, given that poverty rates are high and access to healthcare in general is diminished among the populations most likely to suffer from this particular disorder, there are many more people out there wanting for help than can actually make it to my office.

The Costs Can Be High, Even if the Results Aren't Impressive

You've already learned that the two most common types of practitioners that keloid sufferers visit are dermatologists and surgeons, quite often plastic surgeons.

Those practitioners, of course, don't practice medicine for free and the cost of any competent medical professional's time is likely to be high.

How much could those treatments cost? It can vary according to the market, the practitioner and many other factors, but here are some averages to consider.

Steroid injections are typically among the least expensive treatments, sometimes costing $200 or less, but oftentimes more.

Laser treatments—which don't work for keloids—can cost as much as $5,000 or more.

Home remedies, such as ear bands, cost almost nothing, but are very likely to do either no good or actual harm. They work by cutting off blood flow to the keloid tissue. This is very likely to cut off blood flow to healthy tissue, as well, resulting in necrosis and disfigurement. It's not likely to remove a keloid, in any case.

Surgery, of course, really has no ceiling on how much it costs.

To make the surgical option worse, keloid sufferers that seek it out, to no avail, are likely to have more and more surgeries recommended to them, despite the overall negative outcomes. This racks up huge bills and, in the end, may cause a secondary keloid.

If you are considering the surgical option out of desperation, remember that secondary keloids are sometimes completely untreatable and oftentimes much larger than the primary keloid the surgery was supposed to remove.

If you can, come visit my office but, whatever you do, do not try to have a keloid surgically removed.

Moreover, please do not try home remedies or quack cures. You'll only frustrate yourself and may drive up your medical costs by doing additional damage that needs to be repaired, on top of the costs of what genuinely effective keloid treatments are out there.

Before we go on, it is important to note that there is no group that is immune to keloid disorder.

In an article entitled *Yes ma'am, white people do get keloids*, published on NDSMCObserver.com, writer Katherine Khorey gives a very good example of how a disorder that affects many people can end up being associated with one group so strongly that most people think that the suffering is only experienced by one part of the population, when that may well not be the case.

Disenfranchisement Means Lack of Interest

According to the NAACP, African Americans face some serious hurdles to getting healthcare.

The NAACP points out that, in forty-five states, health insurance companies can discriminate against people if they have pre-existing conditions when they attempt to purchase health insurance directly.

Add that to the higher incidents of chronic medical conditions among African Americans noted above and you can see that there are definitely obstacles in place.

When people don't have healthcare, they're obviously far less likely to visit a doctor on a regular basis. In addition to the way that this can exacerbate potentially deadly conditions, it can also make conditions such as keloid disorder worse for lack of treatment.

Since this significant segment of the population doesn't seek medical treatment in larger numbers, there's less interest in conditions that primarily affect African Americans.

When it comes down to it, healthcare is a business. Research into new treatments, to some degree, is done based on the potential profitability of those treatments.

If the community those treatments is likely to serve most often isn't frequenting healthcare providers in great numbers, it follows that there would be less interest in pursuing them from healthcare providers and pharma companies.

In the end, there just isn't enough lobbying for effective treatments for keloid disorder.

There needs to be an organization that advocates for everyone who suffers from keloid disorder, heritage notwithstanding. That, of course, is what the KRF is set up to do, but it's a long and expensive road to getting where the KRF needs to be, and where the medical community should be in terms of treating this disease.

Lest you think that referencing socio-economic and racial barriers as impediments to research is some empty charge, consider another disease that affects African Americans: sickle cell anemia.

The article *Social Aspects of Sickle Cell Anemia*, available at Biology.Kenyon.Edu, notes that, in the early 1980s, there was approximately $100,000 raised for the study of sickle cell anemia. Contrast this with the millions of dollars raised to study other diseases, such as muscular dystrophy and cystic fibrosis in the same time period, as the article encourages, and the discrepancy is obvious.

There are very real barriers to progress presented to us by preexisting social conditions.

Just as a preexisting medical condition might prevent you from getting necessary treatments covered by an insurance provider, social conditions unfairly separate suffering people from the relief they could, and should, have.

The sooner all of these various walls are torn down the sooner we can advance, in medicine and in so many other ways.

You Can Help

Awareness is a significant advantage in working toward a treatment for any disease or disorder. Consider how effective awareness efforts have been at getting money devoted to research into breast cancer.

Where keloid disorder is concerned, any amount of awareness can go a long way.

If you know someone with keloid disorder, be sure to share what you learn in this book. Let them know about the hazards of the most commonly prescribed treatments and why they should seriously consider alternatives.

If it's possible for them to do so, feel free to refer them to me. I see many patients who suffer this disorder every week and, over the last few years, I've seen over 900. That number continues to climb.

Where finding a treatment for this disorder and getting the medical establishment involved are concerned, knowledge truly is power. The more people who know about this disorder and the more people are willing to talk about it, the more likely it is that something will be done.

As was pointed out, if your physician recommends a treatment that I've already specifically recommended against, consider that I am the only specialist in this field right now.

Just as the lack of a lobby for keloid sufferers has negative impacts on the number of available treatments, the lack of knowledge among physicians impacts the courses of action they recommend.

Every week, I see people who got precisely the wrong treatments, and whose conditions only got worse, sometimes to the point of being untreatable.

By all means, feel free to send me an email or visit my site, http://Keloid212.com, for more information. At the very least, you can get accurate information about your condition, and you're likely to be surprised at what you learn.

More than anything, you'll see that there are many people out there just like you.

In the next chapter, we'll go into greater depth about what's involved in medical research, and the institutional barriers that stand in the way of meaningful progress.

CHAPTER 8

Institutional Barriers Are Very Real

n this chapter, you'll learn:

- That medical research is intricate, expensive and difficult
- That a great deal of funding is needed to complete medical studies
- That some existing treatments have great potential as therapies for keloid disorder
- That getting funding, and approval, for new treatments is exceedingly difficult

We've gone over the work the KRF seeks to do a bit already. We've also gone over some of the challenges it faces.

In this chapter, I'd like to help you to understand what we're really facing in terms of obstacles to finding a cure, and *why* we are facing those obstacles.

What we need to be able to do is to carry out research

into keloid disorder, including its origins, its best treatment options and beyond.

That will entail significant, and potentially expensive, efforts.

For better or worse, medicine is a business. There must be the promise of profitability to secure funding for research, in many cases.

Because keloid disorder tends to affect people who are typically disenfranchised from the healthcare system in general, and because insurance companies don't pay for treatments, there are two obvious obstacles that need to be overcome.

Hopefully, this book will serve to increase overall awareness of keloid disorder.

For the reader's benefit, I'd also like to take some time to make you aware of what researching treatments for keloid disorder would likely entail. It should provide some enlightenment as to the common challenges we face: you, as someone who suffers this disorder; myself, as someone who very much wants to provide relief to patients.

Genetic Research

As you've learned, my background is in oncology. Oncology is a field that has benefited significantly from genetic research.

Such research has allowed modern medicine to develop new treatments for one of the most terrifying and deadly of all diseases: cancer.

You've also learned that keloid disorder shares much in common with cancer.

- Keloid disorder is genetic in its origins, just as is cancer.

- Keloid disorder can be difficult, or nigh impossible to detect in some patients, just like cancer.

- Keloid disorder responds to some chemotherapy drugs, again, just as does cancer.

For anyone who addresses diseases and disorders from a scientific view—which, at least I would hope, includes any competent practitioner of modern medicine—these commonalities are too significant to ignore.

The first point, however, makes genetic research a tool that has enormous utility in gaining an understanding of keloid disorder.

The KRF very much wants to engage in sophisticated and comprehensive genetic research into keloid disorder, but it is not a simple task.

The Basics of Genetic Research

You likely know a bit about genetics, but allow me to give you a broad, layman's overview of how it applies to diseases and disorders and finding treatments for both.

Your genes are, essentially, the blueprints for your body. They dictate how your body will grow, how it will develop and, to a great extent, what sort of difficulties—and advantages—you'll face along the way.

In your body, there are roughly 25,000 genes. Each of those genes uses a code, which we represent using four letters, to determine how the gene should function.

We owe some of our unique qualities to the subtle variations in our genetic code. You may be tall or short, have your father's strong jaw or your mother's lustrous hair. It's all in your blueprint.

Sometimes those small differences between one person's genetic code and the next result in slight, but relatively benign, abnormalities. You may have one leg that's a bit shorter than the other, but that causes you no real handicap. You might be colorblind, prone to early balding or deal with some other issue.

Such problems could be caused by variations such as missing pieces in your genetic code or, in some cases, some additional genetic code that you carry that deviates from the norm.

Sometimes, however, the genetic code becomes altered in a way that is life changing. Such is the case with keloid disorder.

Tracing Your Family History

You might trace the aforementioned strong jaw or lustrous hair back to your father or mother; gifts they passed down to you through the wonders of genetics.

You can also credit them with your keloid disorder, as this disorder is passed down through the genes.

Studies into cancer have shown, over and over again, that some families have a very high rate of cancer among their members. This propensity for developing potentially life-threatening cancers is passed through the genes.

By studying this relationship, medical scientists have been able to devise simple, but potentially life-saving, protocols.

For example, if you are a woman whose mother died of breast cancer, your doctor will most certainly encourage you to keep up with your scheduled mammograms. This is a simple piece of advice, but one that could very well save your life.

If your parents suffered Alzheimer's disease, your doctor will, likewise, encourage you to be conscious of any symptoms that you may exhibit, so potentially useful treatments can be employed before the disease progresses too far.

Further, genetic research can give an even more detailed view of such diseases. One side of a family, for instance, may pass along a propensity to cancer, while members of the other side of your family might have very low rates of cancer.

By performing detailed genetic research into such cases, medical scientists can get down to the root causes of such disorders and, in some instances, develop incredibly useful and effective treatments.

This is what the KRF would like to delve into where keloid disorder is concerned. The same techniques used in other types of genetic research could be eminently useful in learning more about keloid disorder.

By studying families that have the disorder, we could potentially learn which genes carry the disorder and, therefore, how it might be tested for.

By studying members of families that carry the gene, but are unaffected by the disorder, we could potentially discover what triggers it.

Imagine being able to avoid or suppress whatever it is that causes keloid disorder to manifest in a patient!

By studying large populations, we could discover what differs between people who carry this disorder and people who do not.

There is so much potential here that, in fact, the possibilities for creating new treatments are almost as mind-boggling as the sophistication of the science behind genetic research itself.

Sadly, the best genetic research we have right now is simply lineage. If your father, mother or other close relative has keloid disorder, we at least know you're at a higher risk. We cannot tell you how much your risk is increased, nor can we give you a definitive answer as to whether or not you have keloid disorder.

Those answers, as it stands, are ones we can only determine when we see your first keloid develop, and that doesn't have to be the case.

Genetic research is but one goal of the KRF. There are other types of research that would need to be carried out, and they can be very expensive.

Testing the Problem Tissue

Because keloid disorder is a condition that affects the skin, it's logical that studying the skin could lead to breakthroughs.

Studying the keloids themselves, and comparing them to healthy tissue, is precisely the course of action I've suggested to a major NY university as part of a research proposal.

Explaining a bit about how this study will be conducted will help you to develop a better overall understanding of genetic research.

The study will endeavor to gain increased knowledge of the genetic factors involved in this disorder, which are also called the genomics of the disorder by researchers.

To that end, the study will attempt to learn what genetic mutations are involved in the disease process, as well as discovering its biological pathways.

To accomplish this, a study that compares keloid tissue to normal skin tissue could be enormously productive.

Some of the tissue samples would be taken from only one patient. Their normal skin tissue would be compared to their keloid tissue.

Comparisons of tissue taken from different patients, both with and without keloid disorder, would also be performed.

To give you a better idea of the tremendous complexity involved in such studies, consider something you already know about keloids: there are many different types.

The current hypothesis is that each type of keloid—flat, nodular, solitary, multiple, etc.—would have a specific genetic signature associated with it that could provide insight into the cause of the condition.

Comparing the various types of keloid tissue to see how they differ from one to the next, as well as comparing keloid tissue with normal tissue, could yield significant knowledge, and would be part of this work.

The study would also examine tissue samples from an existing databank at the university, expanding the scope of the study.

The tissue samples that would be taken from the databank, because the university is located in New York, have even more potential than you might think at first, simply because of New York's incredibly diverse population.

The tissue bank contains samples from people from all over the world, including Middle Eastern, Asian, European, and African immigrants, as well as people from different areas of the US.

This study would allow researchers to gather detailed genetic data that could be of great value in the fight against keloid disorder.

Remember that, while we do know that keloid is a genetic disorder, we do not yet understand by what process it manifests.

This study could shine a light onto keloid disorder that allows us to expand our vision beyond our current, rather poorly-defined picture of how and why it appears at all.

The specifics of this type of research get very complicated, even compared to other types of genetic research but, to give you a broad outline, here are the types of comparisons that would be conducted:

- Comparisons of different types of keloid tissues obtained from a single patient
- Comparisons of the genetics of keloid tissues to those of normal tissues gathered from a single patient
- Comparisons of keloid tissues gathered from different patients
- Comparisons of normal skin tissues gathered from different patients
- Comparisons of keloid tissue to the genetics of keloid tissues stored in the skin data bank
- Comparisons of normal skin from patients to normal skin in the skin sample databank
- Comparisons of keloid tissue from this study to keloid studies published from around the world

These types of comparisons allow us to see the differences in the genetics between healthy and keloid tissues from a broad selection of donors.

This could potentially provide the missing pieces of information that would finally allow medical science to develop a truly comprehensive knowledge of keloid disorder.

While this study would only be gathering new samples from African American participants who have a positive family history of keloid, the possibility of using the tremendous library of tissue samples increases the scope of the science enormously. The impact of that on the comprehensiveness of the study cannot be overstated.

At this point, if you've been an attentive reader, you will know that this research is not without some risk to the patient. Taking a tissue sample requires a biopsy which, of course, requires that tissue be removed from keloids and from areas of healthy skin.

That carries the risk of keloid formation. Patients that elect to participate in this study will be informed of that risk. This is basic medical ethics.

These patients, however, may end up contributing to significant advances in our understanding of keloid disorder. Their contributions could end up providing the foundational genetic knowledge doctors will require to develop treatments.

Beyond that, the tales that the genes of keloid sufferers have to tell may inform us of better ways to assess risk.

Being able to develop new treatments as a result of this research would change many lives.

Being able to develop comprehensive and accurate ways to test for keloid disorder may prevent it from ever having an impact on the life of someone who it may have otherwise devastated.

This might seem like something of a dream, and for many keloid sufferers, the results this study could potentially yield are, indeed, the type of things they dream about.

By harnessing the incredible investigatory powers that science has to offer, the knowledge, dedication and creativity of physicians and the courage of patients willing to participate in the study, we could make tests, treatments and possibly even a cure for keloid disorder a reality.

If this study sounds like one that you might be interested in participating in, and if you're of African American heritage with a positive family history of keloid disorder, then please do contact my office. Contact information is given in the final chapter of the book.

Genetic tissue analysis and comparison is one of the most innovative and advanced areas of medical research. You could be a part of it.

Clinical Trials

We did touch on clinical trials already, but understanding them to a greater depth will give you a better idea of why it's so difficult to get them up and running without proper support.

Clinical trials allow doctors to utilize and assess the effectiveness of various treatments in a controlled setting.

They require tremendous resources; they require significant amounts of funding. They must be approved and monitored, as well, by a body qualified to assess the safety of the trial.

Getting that approval, as you're going to learn, can mean the difference between hope and despair, both for patients and for the doctors that want more than anything to be able to offer them comfort, treatment and, ultimately, a cure for their condition.

A clinical trial is a very controlled and tightly-monitored

application of a potential treatment for a disease or disorder. It requires volunteers that are willing to be test subjects for the treatment.

There are some widely-held misconceptions about these trials that we should address.

The trials are designed to be as safe as possible, first and foremost. Patients are informed as to the risks involved and, if they are not comfortable with those risks, they are certainly under no obligation to participate.

In fact, it's not too much to say that the patients who participate in such treatments are, though uncredited for it, heroes for other people who end up benefitting from the outcomes of successful trials.

In a clinical trial, the patients participating get treatments that have been developed based on research into a condition that they suffer.

For instance, if genetic research into keloid disorder were to yield an identifiable cause of the disease and, further, a potential way to suppress that cause, the method of offering that to the patient would be tested during the course of the trial.

These trials can be carried out in a number of different venues. Medical schools, government organizations and many other institutions serve as the proving grounds for new and innovative treatments, in many cases.

The trials can also be funded by a number of different organizations. A university might fund them, or a pharmaceutical company might put their significant financial resources behind a study.

The people that actually conduct the study can include a number of different medical professionals. If a new chemotherapy treatment were being tried for keloid disorder, for instance, doctors might provide the treatment to patients, assisted by nurses and other medical staff.

Clinical trials vary significantly in the amount of time involved. If a treatment was expected to take quite a long time to show results, the study could theoretically go on for months or years.

Where keloid disorder is concerned, the goals of such a trial would be in line with the goals of most clinical trials. They might include:

- Developing ways to screen for the disorder
- Developing drug therapies that can prevent or treat the disorder
- Improving the treatments utilized on existing keloids to offer better methods of removing or reducing lesions
- Developing ways to improve the quality of life for keloid sufferers

You may have heard studies of various types—oftentimes polls—faulted for taking too small a sample. The benefits of having a large group of people to study is significant where clinical trials are concerned.

Ideally, a clinical trial conducted by the KRF would involve a significant number of patients, which would allow for the gathering of more useful data than could be obtained from a smaller number of participants.

Even Existing Treatments Could Benefit

Right now, one of the most common treatments ordered for keloid disorder is steroid injection. As was pointed out earlier, no one knows what the proper dosage is for using steroids to treat keloids.

These are the types of questions that clinical trials could answer. Aside from working out truly innovative and completely new treatment options, they can be employed to improve existing treatments.

Just for a moment, consider how strange it is to say what was just stated about steroid treatments. Imagine going to three different doctors to get treatment for a bacterial infection and being prescribed three different dosages of an antibiotic. Not because the physicians had different opinions, but because they just didn't know how much to give you.

This is the type of situation keloid sufferers deal with every day, and it doesn't need to be this way.

The cure to the lack of knowledge in the medical community is research, but there are barriers to making that happen.

Lack of Interest Equals Lack of Therapies

As a casual reader, you might not be all that interested in reviewing medical studies and the records of drugs that have been submitted to the FDA for the treatment of keloids.

Whenever I go to any of the large sites that catalog medical studies, I'm dismayed at the lack of research into keloids. The sheer absence of any work in this regard is shocking.

Moreover, the number of drugs that have been submitted to the FDA for approval as treatments for keloids is even more telling.

How many have been submitted?

Zero.

I have theories on this matter, and I'd like to share them with you.

First, as I've stated, African Americans are disproportionately affected by keloid disorder. Though the US may be the leading nation in terms of medical research, African Americans just do not have sufficient enough a voice to pressure the medical industry, and that makes a huge difference in terms of how much research has been done and how much is likely to be done. No pressure, in short, equals no research.

On my own part, I have struggled to reach out to various groups to foster an interest in this condition. In fact, I have done so over and over again.

The only institution that showed any real interest was a not-for-profit university located in New York City.

Keloid disorder, like any other medical condition, cannot be treated, or even studied, by one person alone. It takes an army to do the type of research required to develop hypotheses into useful theories that can further be turned into practical and efficacious treatments.

There Is Always Frustration

Let me share with you a frustrating example of how institutional resistance can hinder progress.

Because my background is in oncology, I've dedicated a great deal of my life and my practice to treating people suffering with cancer.

Based on my experiences, I developed a research protocol for using a very innovative anti-cancer drug as a treatment for keloid disorder. This was based on my long experience and, more importantly, on the mechanism of action of this drug.

This protocol was designed for the patients with the worst cases of keloid disorder. You might be among them. If you're not, I encourage you to see my website and YouTube pages for some idea of how severe this disorder can get.

These patients have no other recourse available to them through modern medicine. They are, quite literally, with their backs against the wall in this regard.

The FDA blocked me. They said the treatment used a drug that was unsafe. Let's return again to a point that was made earlier, because it is particularly relevant here.

Those patients who are so unfortunate as to be in this situation have no alternative. Do not for one moment think that, simply because their tumors are benign, that their lesions aren't capable of quite literally destroying their quality of life.

Some of these patients live their lives in a way that we might associate with someone unfortunate enough to have been born with a deformity in a less enlightened era. They cover themselves with hoodies, wigs or, if they're very lucky, their hair is long and thick enough to cover their disfigured ears and faces.

Some of them have keloids to such an extent that they do not enjoy the full range of motion their joints should provide.

Some of them suffer constant pain. In some cases the pain is enough to cause sleep disruptions.

Patients with particularly large keloids may also suffer with other accompanying problems, such as obstructed ear canals that diminish their hearing.

In short, those patients who would have been appropriate candidates for this type of treatment might not be suffering from a deadly condition, but they are most certainly suffering from one that has significant impacts on their quality of life.

I went back and forth with the FDA about this study and did my best to make it happen. Once again, however, one person cannot successfully fight this war and, when a very large institution stands in the way of what could provide genuine progress toward finding more effective treatments, there is seemingly little that can be done.

It's important to keep in mind what an impression some interest from a larger number of physicians could make.

Rather than I, alone, standing in front of an FDA board asking for approval, it would mean more doctors, which lends more credibility to the proposed treatment, and a greater chance that it would be approved.

I have tried to get other doctors engaged; doctors whose area of expertise, experience, positions and reputations would have been very helpful. I received no help.

It takes many people to conduct a study, a great deal of money to fund it and large institutions to back it up.

Keeping Discouragement at Bay

This chapter, most certainly, has not been one that's likely to leave you with a great deal of hope, but this has always been the challenge in any medical endeavor.

Put simply, medicine is always a losing battle. Even in this age of advanced genetic therapies, drugs that are targeted to specific conditions and other modern treatments and cures, doctors fight a battle that is oftentimes waged against conditions that have been persistent issues for decades, centuries, even millennia.

People die every day from infections. People die from vitamin deficiencies, scurvy, appendicitis and other treatable conditions.

This should not dissuade us from treating those conditions when we can, and it does not.

Just as there are always problems in finding ways to offer comfort and cures to those afflicted with medical issues, there have always been people willing to buck the mainstream, to demand that neglected conditions be addressed and that continue on, despite having to fight vigorously for every inch of ground gained.

Let's go back to that question of profitability in medicine, because it is relevant to this discussion.

Profitability and Medicine

In a CNN blog from 2013 entitled *U.S health care's dangerous profit fixation* by Russell J. Andrews, a neurosurgeon, the author makes a very salient point.

> "*In essence, we have transformed health care in the U.S. into an industry whose goal is to be profitable, and the health of the patient is not really in the equation.*" (Andrews 2013)

Dr. Andres is precisely right in his point, but the influence of the profit motive extends far beyond the delivery of healthcare.

Over the years, treatments have become business, to be certain, but research has become business, as well.

Unfortunately for the people who suffer with it, keloid disorder has not proven to be profitable for the massive business interests that, to a great degree, guide the direction of medical research in this nation.

A physician who loves his or her art lives for, as the aforementioned author put it, the "joy" that comes with being able to heal someone who visits you for care.

There is quite simply nothing like that joy. Being able to

offer relief to someone who is in desperate need of it; being able to correct a disfigurement that has caused untold psychological and social suffering: those things are truly what makes the endless toil of medicine worth every moment spent practicing it.

But that joy and, more importantly, the ability to truly care for patients from which it flows, are not the things that motivate a great deal of research and development today.

For a dermatologist, it's much easier to pop into the office, spend fifteen or twenty minutes giving a Botox injection and to collect a healthy sum than it is to apply their efforts to a long-term treatment for keloid disorder.

For a plastic surgeon, performing a simple removal of a keloid seems easy enough. When those patients come back, more disfigured than ever, more surgeries mean more profits, of course.

That's not to say that these practitioners are motivated entirely by profit, but it does illustrate a point.

In getting the kind of research that's required to develop an effective treatment for keloid disorder, the current situation is one where we find ourselves with hat in hand.

Hopefully, someone with deep pockets will step forward and offer to shine a spotlight on this disorder and all the suffering it causes.

Hopefully, someone who is already in the spotlight, such as a celebrity, will come forward and discuss experiences they may have had with keloid disorder.

As it stands, however, there is too little funding to conduct the kind of research that's required.

As we discussed in an earlier chapter, this disorder also happens to mainly affect a population that is typically on the fringes of the medical community. Without the promise of large profits, which seem unlikely from that community, it may be a very difficult fight to get the funding that is needed.

I cannot win this fight on my own, but I will keep fighting. I advocate for awareness and the development of new treatments. I try to get my colleagues involved. I try to get institutions involved. I approach the FDA with new treatments.

I cannot do this on my own, but I will keep at it and, I hope, some others with the clout and financial wherewithal to make this fight productive will come forward to help, as well.

An Endless Cycle that Could Be Stopped

There is a genuine need for effective treatments for keloid disorder.

Right now, someone is developing their first keloid and it pains me to think that they're also considering having it cut out, which is only going to exacerbate their condition.

Right now, someone is losing sleep because their keloid itches and burns to the point of being maddening.

Right now, someone is being recommended as a candidate for radiation therapy. That therapy will not help them, and it may well end up killing them, due to resulting cancer.

Right now, someone is afraid to be physically intimate because they hate the way their body looks.

A teenager is being ostracized and bullied because of keloids on their face or ears.

Someone is being passed over for a job, simply because their condition makes them look unhealthy and diseased, even though they may be genuinely healthy and fit.

It doesn't need to be this way, but it is. Profit is, indeed, a petty thing compared to all this suffering.

But I and others involved in the KRF will keep fighting, as doctors always have, even though the battle may be hard and the world deaf to it even being waged.

CHAPTER 9

You Could Play a Role in Helping to Raise Awareness

I n this chapter, you'll learn that:

- People can make a difference in influencing the medical community

- There are good doctors out there that want to help

- There are ways that you could help fight keloid disorder

- You don't have to make a huge impact on the medical community to make a meaningful difference

Where raising awareness of medical conditions is concerned, there is likely no disease that comes so readily to mind as does breast cancer, and for good reason.

Breast cancer awareness efforts have combined techniques from a diverse array of sources. Where medicine is concerned, physicians encourage women to get mammograms and inform them of the increased survival rates associated with the early detection of cancers.

Socially, breast cancer awareness efforts have borrowed heavily from the marketing practices used by advertising agencies, salespeople and other professionals who make their living persuading people to get engaged with products and ideas.

There's a complex intertwining of symbols, emotions, desires and other factors that contribute to making breast cancer such a recognizable brand. The term "brand" is not used frivolously here, and it speaks to a powerful and admirable effort on the part of those who have worked so hard to raise awareness of breast cancer. Branding is a powerful tool in raising awareness of any condition, and it could most certainly play a role in raising the awareness of keloid disorder.

To date, however, keloid disorder is foiled in this regard due to several factors:

- It is not commonly known or understood
- Even the medical community lacks comprehensive knowledge of the disorder
- It principally affects an already marginalized segment of the population
- It is not a deadly condition

We've discussed the preceding sources of frustration at length already, so let's take a different perspective here. Let's talk about how the awareness of keloid disorder could be increased by a similar branding campaign to that used so effectively to promote breast cancer awareness and research.

People Have to Know What it Is

First and foremost among the challenges to raising aware-ness of keloid disorder is the simple fact that most people don't know what it is or how it affects people.

Additionally, keep in mind that gaining public support for the sufferers of this disorder is an uphill battle. Where the sufferers of breast cancer face a potentially mortal illness, keloid sufferers aren't facing death itself.

That doesn't mean that there isn't a way to convey the urgency of this condition. Consider what you've learned already.

- Some keloid sufferers face serious impacts, such as hearing impairment or diminished mobility in their limbs, due to their condition

- Keloid sufferers sometimes endure horrible self-es-teem issues due to the disfiguring nature of keloids

- Keloid sufferers face devastating social impacts as a result of their appearance

- Keloid sufferers may have a hard time finding a job due to their appearance

These are all very real, very immediate impacts of this disorder. In the most basic terms, when someone has keloid disorder, they are also suffering. They may not be suffering the prospect of their own death, but they are suffering con-sequences that are just as immediate: economic, social and psychological, in addition to their physical suffering.

Raising awareness of what this disorder is and how it affects people, beyond the keloids themselves, could go a long way toward pressuring the medical community to pay more attention to the condition and those that suffer from it.

If you are a keloid sufferer, the obvious course of action is to explain your condition should the opportunity arise. It's never pleasant to draw attention to an issue that likely already causes you significant distress. However, each time that you do so, and each time someone stops for a moment and learns from you, means that there's one more person who knows about the disorder, its impacts and how it affects someone they know, or a stranger that they just happened to run into.

This has the effect of humanizing the disorder. Remember that, when people think of breast cancer, they don't think of tumors. They most likely think of how it could affect someone they know; someone they love.

That is how keloid disorder has to be framed for the public at large.

Tying Keloid to a Population

As we've gone over in some detail, keloid disorder principally affects the African American population.

Because that population enjoys less contact with the healthcare system, myriad problems, which we've also discussed, present themselves when trying to raise awareness of keloid disorder.

However, keloid disorder does not exclusively affect the African American population. In addition to this fact, while there are significant racial barriers, both social and institutional, that must be overcome, there has also been a great deal of progress made over the years, upon which awareness efforts could capitalize.

Breast cancer awareness benefitted from the fact that it

can be so closely tied to the overall issue of women's health. Every woman is someone's friend, partner, sister, mother, grandmother and so forth. This puts a human face on breast cancer and makes it readily apparent what a threat it is to everyone.

Everyone with keloid disorder is a friend, sister, brother, mother, father, as well. While this is a condition that principally affects African Americans, it does affect everyone and, what's more, it could affect anyone at any time. Remember: many people have this disorder and don't even find out until later in life, to devastating effect.

Therefore, it seems that the disorder can be humanized and personalized rather easily, if people were more aware of it.

This is a challenge, but not an insurmountable one.

As we've discussed already, there are Internet groups where people who suffer this disorder discuss their experiences. Social media presents an opportunity to do much the same.

Every time a meme is shared, a story posted and so forth, there's a chance that someone who formerly knew nothing about keloid disorder will become aware of its existence and, moreover, that they may share that knowledge with others.

There needs to be a movement of some sort if we are to address keloid disorder as the serious medical issue it is.

There needs to be a movement soon, in fact, because far too many people are suffering with a disorder that, given modern medicine's capabilities where research and the development of cures are concerned, should be curable.

Share your stories. Share your experiences. In doing so, you help to remove the impression that keloid disorder is something that affects some other people, somewhere else and you remind people that it affects individuals from all walks of life.

As part of raising awareness, it's important to let people know which treatment options work and which do not.

Building Awareness of What Doesn't Work Matters

Consider how much good has been done for women by making them more aware of the value of mammograms. By testing for the presence of cancer on a regular basis, physicians can increase the likelihood that any ordered treatments will be effective and thus, that the patient will survive.

Persuading women to get regular mammograms is a goal in and of itself, but it's not the ultimate goal. The ultimate goal is to make sure that women who require them have ready access to effective treatments for any cancer that's detected.

There needs to be a similar movement for keloid sufferers. There needs to be a movement to make them aware that getting checked for the condition—as much as doing so is possible—is imperative toward achieving the best outcomes.

That first step would entail letting people know about:

- The inherited nature of keloid disorder
- The fact that sufferers may not know they have it until it actually manifests
- The fact that precautions can be taken to avoid making it worse, if it already has manifested

Consider the mammogram example again, and its relationship to providing access to proven, science-based treatments.

When a woman gets a mammogram, she's already in contact with qualified, knowledgeable professionals who practice effective medicine. Nonetheless, making women aware of the real, tested options for treatment is a challenge, and there are people out there willing to lead cancer patients astray for a profit.

The FDA maintains a webpage where they document fake cancer cures. Certainly, there are any number of quacks out there offering fake cures for keloid disorder and, if you're so inclined, you can do a web search and see a lot of pages advertising such cures for yourself.

Keloid sufferers, in this regard, face a double threat.

While a woman who has breast cancer, and whose cancer is detected early, will be working with physicians who can offer her the best available treatments, the medical professionals that keloid sufferers are in contact with may offer precisely the *wrong* treatments.

Moreover, they will do so with the incredible authority that comes with carrying the title of Medical Doctor.

This is not quackery. Again, the plastic surgeons and dermatologists who offer treatments—the wrong treatments—for keloid disorder are doing their best. They're using the tools and knowledge available to them and trying to provide a positive outcome for their patient.

They're not being deceitful, as a quack would be. They're merely misguided and, because of that, they end up doing more harm than good.

Keloid disorder sufferers, unfortunately, must be made aware of a very painful truth.

- There are no tests that can further illuminate their condition

- There are no drugs that are readily available for treatment
- There are no surgeries that can simply cut out the keloid without a severe risk of recurrence

For the sufferers of cancer and many other dangerous conditions, the process of getting treatment starts with becoming aware of the disease, proceeds through consultations with physicians to determine the best course of action and relies on the application of proven treatments to cure, or at least control, the disease.

Keloid sufferers, sadly, must rely on patience more than anything else. A hasty visit to a plastic surgeon will only make the condition worse. Likewise, heading to a dermatologist is likely to be of little, if any, benefit.

Remember that you can always encourage a keloid sufferer to contact me. Even if they are unable to get to my clinic, I can at least impart to them what I know about the condition and let them know what kind of treatment options are out there.

You can always refer them to my site or my YouTube videos so they can see other patient's stories and, just as importantly, learn about the dangers of pursuing the wrong courses of treatment.

Hopefully, seeing that information, they'll know not to go to legitimate practitioners who are misguided as to the effective treatments for keloid disorder and, most certainly, not to waste their money on quack cures that will do nothing but lighten their wallets and frustrate their hopes.

There is a more significant issue here than misguided physicians or quack cures. There are some practitioners who advertise themselves as being able to provide relief from keloids specifically, oftentimes using plastic surgery.

As you've learned, and should remember: plastic surgery will not work for keloids, no matter how many times you're told differently.

Plastic surgery is not the answer. Going to a plastic surgeon is simply setting yourself up for a terrible outcome.

A Somewhat Flooded Market

There are many different awareness efforts, covering a huge variety of different illnesses.

As an example of this, consider the colored ribbons that are employed as a way to brand awareness efforts.

Currently, there are so many awareness efforts that a particular color can represent any of a number of different conditions. To reference breast cancer again, it's a mark of the success of that awareness effort that most people seeing a pink ribbon will likely think of breast cancer before anything else.

According to DisabledWorld.com, the pink ribbon also stands for birth parents and nursing mothers.

What does this mean? Simply that there are so many different awareness efforts that standing out can be a problem for any one group trying to increase research into a particular condition.

While this is an uphill battle, it is one that is worth fighting and, if one form of branding—awareness ribbons, etc.— is not likely to work, that shouldn't stop keloid sufferers and medical professionals from trying to raise general awareness of the condition.

Imagine how much easier life would have been for at least a portion of severe keloid sufferers if they'd known:

- About the hereditary nature of keloid disorder
- About what kind of procedures—e.g. ear piercing—might not be suitable choices for them
- About how certain treatments would exacerbate their keloids
- About how there is an organization, the KRF, that actively seeks to provide accurate information about keloid disorder

It would be nice, certainly, if keloid disorder got the same level of attention as some other conditions. Simply because that may not be the case right now does not mean that we should stop trying to inform people.

Those of us empowered with accurate information about keloid disorder—including you, having read this book—should seek to spread it wherever possible. Doing so is only for the better.

How You Can Get Involved

If you do want to get involved with helping us find treatments for keloid disorder, I urge you to take a look at the Keloid Research Foundation site at KeloidResearchFoundation.org.

On that site, you'll find our Keloid Encounter page, where we post the true stories of patients coping with keloid disorder.

Each of these stories can help you to better understand keloid disorder, even if you don't suffer from it yourself. It's also a great educational resource if you do suffer from keloid disorder and need to provide information for friends, coworkers and others who may inquire about your condition.

Of course, if you should happen to come across someone who has no knowledge whatsoever of the disorder and want to provide them with an understanding of what keloid disorder means for the people who suffer with it, the Encounters section of the KRF website is an excellent resource to offer them.

As an aside, the KRF site also contains information on how interested persons can participate in studies that may provide us with the knowledge we need to make meaningful progress toward more effective treatments for keloid disorder. Should one of the people you refer to the page want to enroll, it would only be beneficial.

Keep Spreading the Word

Remember that anything you can do to inform people of your condition, if you're a keloid sufferer, or of keloid disorder in general if you don't have it yourself, does help.

You might be surprised at how many people you meet who do have, to some degree or another, keloid disorder. Those who haven't suffered significant amounts of keloid growth may never have bothered to have their keloids checked out by a physician. Or, if they did, the keloid may have simply been regarded as a minor problem and not addressed.

A bit of awareness might help such individuals to avoid making mistakes that could lead to a much larger keloid, and encourage them to exercise caution where their children are concerned.

Researching keloid disorder will require a great deal of

money and work. Neither of those things will be lent to the effort unless the entities that control those resources are pressured by the public.

Any amount of awareness you can raise helps, so please make an effort to do so.

Even encouraging people to read this book will help, and please ask people to do so if you get the chance.

Chapter 10

Your Insurance Might Not Cover Your Treatments

n this chapter you'll learn:

- How finances are too often struggles for people who need competent medical care
- That it's very likely that your insurance will *not* cover keloid treatment
- That you may have to pursue other options
- Some tips for dealing with insurance issues

Health insurance is far from perfect, and oftentimes doesn't even reach the much lower bar of simple adequacy.

Since the passage of the Affordable Care Act, it's likely that the vast majority of people reading this book have some form of health coverage.

Unfortunately, it's also likely that your insurance won't cover keloid treatments.

Medicaid and Medicare

If you qualify under income requirements or are retired, you most likely have Medicaid or Medicare coverage.

Unfortunately, it's unlikely that any keloid treatments will be covered by either of these public medical programs. Remember: keloid disorder is considered to be a cosmetic disorder, and these forms of insurance do not cover cosmetic disorders.

There may be an exception if your keloid is causing you some level of disability, such as motion impairment. There also may be an exception if your keloid treatments are medical necessities.

In either case, you'll have to contact whichever agency is responsible for your coverage and speak to a representative. If you visit a physician, they may be able to document the issues that you face because of your keloid disorder and get some procedures covered as medical necessities.

Remember, however, that getting the wrong procedures covered by your insurance is going to do you no good in the long run. We've gone over the procedures that I use. Please take that information into account before you consider pursuing any others, as they may worsen your keloids.

Private Insurance

Private insurance varies significantly from one policy to another in terms of what it covers. In any case, it's highly unlikely that your private insurance policy covers cosmetic procedures, and that's likely how keloid treatments will be classified.

As is the case with public insurance, you'll have to contact your provider to determine whether or not your insurance will pay for keloid treatments.

If not, you'll have to pay out of pocket, and this makes good decisions imperative.

Paying Out of Pocket

Most people seeking keloid treatments will have to pay for those treatments out of their own pockets.

Given what you know about ineffective treatments, paying for the wrong treatments is, in fact, rather adding insult to injury.

If you're going to pursue keloid treatments, planning ahead is a good idea, and I'd like to address the usual pattern of treatment that people go through to drive that point home.

Perhaps your doctor can get your keloid treatments covered by your insurance, or perhaps you find a way to pay for them yourself.

You might go in to your provider, quite naturally wanting to get rid of the keloid as soon as possible.

All the while, you're pursuing a course of action that's going to either do nothing or do real damage.

In the end, you're also going to get a bill for it, possibly a hefty one.

Patience is very much a virtue if you're a keloid sufferer.

Remember that, unless you're within range of my clinic, your only treatment options are quite possibly the worst courses of action. Don't panic about your keloid disorder.

You can get in touch with me to talk about the issue and see if there's a way that you can receive treatments. You'll find plenty of doctors offering keloid treatment on their websites, some of them are likely close to where you live.

I am, however, the only doctor that specializes in treating this condition in North America. Good physicians will warn you that, if you go in to have a keloid surgically removed, there's a risk that you might develop a worse keloid at the site of the surgery. Understand that not only is there a risk, but there is an unacceptably high risk that you're going to develop a more visible lesion.

In fact, you will *almost certainly* develop another keloid.

Don't cross your fingers and start running your credit card to pay for plastic surgery for keloids. If you're hoping the odds are in your favor and the surgery will end up permanently removing your keloid, remember that you'd be much better off betting that your keloid will come back.

It's only a matter of time before it does, in all likelihood, and it will be worse when it returns.

Getting Information on Treatments

Considering that you're likely to have to pay for keloid treatments from your own pocket, the best course of action is to consult with a physician and get an idea of the costs involved.

You can contact my office to learn more about treatments. I emphasize non-surgical treatments. They take time. One of the things that makes people in desperate straits lean toward surgery is the immediacy of the procedure. "Cut it out!" must be the cry of anyone who finds that they have something unwanted, benign or otherwise, on their bodies.

I wish I could tell you that there were other doctors in North America who specialize in this disorder. I cannot, however and, unfortunate as that may be, it is the truth.

Some Good News

It is hard, when discussing a disorder that causes so much misery, and for which there are so few treatment options, to find the occasional bright side.

I can, however, at least offer you some numbers to work with. I do believe that, in so many ways, knowledge is power.

Knowing what to expect financially is as important as knowing what to expect physically when seeking medical treatments. To offer you the advantage of the former, here are some prices from my own practice.

My services are broken into two categories: the initial consultation and following visits and the charges for specific treatments.

The first visit and consultation will cost $250. Subsequent visits cost $150.

The cost of the treatments themselves cannot be offered so plainly, as they may vary considerably between one patient and the next.

The cost of treatment will depend upon the extent of the treatments required, which will depend upon the severity and spread of your keloids.

I can, however, discuss your treatment options and costs with you during the initial consultation. In the following chapter, I will provide you with detailed contact information and the procedure for sending me information about your condition.

Don't Be Impulsive

As a final word, let me caution you again against impulsive action regarding your keloids.

The job of a physician is to develop knowledge and understanding and to use the tools that medical science provides to alleviate suffering.

No such professional likes to see good people spending good money on bad treatments.

Please, if you have questions about your keloid disorder and you're considering visiting a doctor and having a procedure done, whether you found them online or otherwise, consult with me first.

Remember that holding off on any medical procedure might be a better option than getting the wrong procedure performed.

I would certainly prefer that you contact me before you make a bad decision. Even if I cannot treat you at my practice, I can at least offer you good information that may spare you from your condition getting worse and your wallet being made lighter to no useful end.

CHAPTER 11

I Am Here to Help:
How to Get in Touch

My practice is located in New York, NY. If you're located nearby, I invite you to schedule a consultation visit.

You can also contact me via email. I will give detailed instructions on doing so below.

If You've Already Received Treatment

It's often true that, when patients feel that they've taken the wrong course of action with a treatment or in attending to their health in general, they fear being admonished by their doctor.

You can safely let go of that fear. If you've received improper treatment for your keloids already—even after having read this book—do not hesitate to get in touch.

Many of my patients come to me having already suffered improper treatments. Their conditions got worse and, in many cases, they likely feared that their condition was untreatable.

I'm sad to say that, in some instances, that was precisely the case and that there was little that could be done to treat their keloids.

Not all instances turned out so poorly, however, and there are cases where people came in to my practice after enduring many failed treatments and enjoyed excellent results.

You can see examples of such patients on my website and YouTube channel. Links are provided below.

In those videos, you'll often hear about how patients tried many different types of treatments before visiting my clinic. Sometimes, in the interim between these treatments and visiting me, the patients had entirely given up hope.

Don't give up hope, whatever you do.

Even though there may be a lot of work to be done in finding treatments for keloid disorder, there are those of us in the medical community who are more than willing to do that work and who only need to secure the proper funding and resources to begin.

Take a Look at My Results

To get an overview of the treatments I offer, and some of the results I've been able to achieve, go to Keloid212.com to visit my site.

You'll find many different videos that detail the stories of some of my patients, that show their lesions and that describe the types of treatments they received from me, along with the results I was able to achieve.

Some of these videos may bring you significant hope, and justly so. I only wish there were more doctors specializing in keloid disorder.

As you'll hear from some of my patients, pain, itching and burning are common symptoms of keloid disorder. These can also be symptoms of some genuinely dangerous skin conditions, so be sure to have any suspected keloids you might find checked out by a qualified physician.

I would recommend that you not pursue plastic surgery, however, and it very well may be suggested to you as a remedy. As you've learned, plastic surgery seldom offers any good outcome for keloid patients.

How to Contact Me

You can download a form from http://keloid212.com/ra.php to request a consultation from me.

You will need to provide the following information on the form before I can schedule a consultation.

- The reason you're asking for a consultation
- How long you've had a keloid and what age you were when you first noticed it
- Whether there has been any change in the lesion, its growth rate or shape
- If you've had surgery on the keloid and, if so, when
- If you've ever received steroid injections and, if so, when
- If you've ever had radiation treatments and, if so, when
- If you have received other treatments and, if so, when
- If you've ever been diagnosed with skin cancer or Melanoma

- Whether you have a family history of keloid disorder
- If you have any other disorders
- If you're currently taking any medications
- Any other relevant information you might want to include about the keloid

I'm providing this here because it might help you to be better organized when you download the form and start to fill it out. If you have everything beforehand, it seems more likely that you will reach out and I am here to help, so I wish to encourage you to contact me and to make doing so as easy as possible.

You can also make an appointment with me from the aforementioned address, which will be confirmed via email. If this makes it easier for you to manage your appointment, then please take advantage of the option.

Emailing for a First Appointment

For your first contact, please send an email along with the consultation request form. That email should contain images of any keloids you have.

The images help me to give you a better assessment of your condition, and how we might work toward improving it.

Hesitating? Don't

There are many reasons why people hesitate to contact a physician about a condition. Here are some things to consider if you're hesitating about contacting me.

What if my condition isn't treatable?

This is a possibility, certainly. The thing to keep in mind is that you won't know until you get a consultation. The worst case scenario is not that your condition cannot be treated. The worst case scenario is that it can be treated, but that your hesitation prevents you from getting effective treatment.

What if my keloid is something worse?

If you have not been diagnosed with keloid disorder and have self-diagnosed a growing, changing or new lesion on your skin, then you must get to a doctor immediately. Skin cancers are among the deadliest of all cancers and no one—not even a physician—is capable of accurate self-diagnosis.

In all cases, if you see something new or a change in an existing lesion on your skin, please, schedule an appointment with a qualified medical practitioner to get it examined. It may very well save your life.

What if I can't afford treatment?

The only way to get an idea of how much your treatments will cost is through a consultation. Again, even physicians need to conduct an examination before really knowing which course of treatment will be required.

What if my only payment method is insurance?

Unfortunately, we do not accept insurance. Whether or not you receive reimbursement will depend upon your provider. We will give you records of your treatment that you can submit to seek reimbursement, but we have no control over whether or not any claim you file with your insurer will be paid.

What if I cannot get to New York?

I do not provide referrals and only work out of my own offices in New York. However, I still encourage you to take advantage of the information on my website, to educate yourself and to contact a dermatologist about your keloids.

My Contact Information

Here are my contact details.

Mailing Address

Michael H. Tirgan, M.D.
23 West 73rd Street, Suite GD
New York, NY 10023

Telephone:

(212) 874-4200

Email:

DrTirgan@Gmail.com

Google+:

https://plus.google.com/u/0/106284173669049752670/about

YouTube Channel:

https://www.youtube.com/user/DrTirgan

The Keloid Research Foundation:

http://www.KeloidResearchFoundation.org/

Thank You

I wish to thank you for reading this book. I hope it has helped you to learn more about keloid disorder, whether or not you suffer from it personally.

I also hope it will encourage you to avoid treatments that are likely to make your keloids worse and to seek treatments that may help.

If you're so inclined, please spread the word about keloid disorder, and help to shine a light where there exists too much ignorance at present.

It is by speaking up and speaking out that those who suffer from keloid disorder and those close to them are likely to get the attention of the medical community and, hopefully, the pharmaceutical companies and other entities that are financially more than capable of funding the research required to work toward better methods of detecting, and treating, this disorder.

While your insurance company and even, perhaps, your physician will tell you that keloid disorder is cosmetic, I disagree. It is far more than that and, even though it might be a very difficult and long road to getting there, I will continue to work toward conducting better research, devising better treatments and, hopefully, offering keloid sufferers a better quality of life.

I hope that you will join me in this and, if you're located close enough to New York and want to schedule a consultation, please reach out.

Michael H. Tirgan, M.D.

Bibliography

Andrews, Russell J. 2013. *U.S. health care's dangerous profit fixation.* 07 11. http://globalpublicsquare.blogs.cnn.com/2013/07/11/u-s-health-cares-dangerous-profit-fixation/.

Bhate, K, Williams, HC. 2013. *Epidemiology of acne vulgaris.* 03. http://www.ncbi.nlm.nih.gov/pubmed/23210645.

celeste2. 2010. *I Have Keloid Scars.* 05 06. http://www.experienceproject.com/stories/Have-Keloid-Scars/1021557.

Disabled World. n.d. *Awareness Ribbons Chart: Color & Meaning of Awareness Ribbon Causes.* http://www.disabled-world.com/disability/awareness/ribbons.php.

Earth Clinic. 2015. *Natural Treatment for Keloid Scars.* 07 14. http://www.earthclinic.com/cures/keloid_scar.html.

Kenyon College. n.d. *Social Aspects of Sickle Cell Anemia.* http://biology.kenyon.edu/slonc/gene-web/sickle_cell_project/SocialAspects.html.

Khorey, Katherine. 2008. *Yes ma'am, white people do get keroids.* 09 17. http://ndsmcobserver.com/2008/09/yes-maam-white-people-do-get-keroids/.

NAACP. n.d. *http://www.naacp.org/pages/health-care-fact-sheet.* http://www.naacp.org/pages/health-care-fact-sheet.

Olaitan, Peter B, Victoria Odensina, Samuel Ademola, Solomon O Fadiora, and Odunayo M and Reichenberger, Ernst J Oluwatosin. 2014. *Recruitment of Yoruba families from Nigeria for genetic research: experience from a multisite keloid study.* 09 02. http://www.biomedcentral.com/1472-6939/15/65.

Ressler-Culp, Tara. 2014. *Why Racism Is A Public Health Issue.* 02 03. http://thinkprogress.org/health/2014/02/03/3239101/racism-public-health-issue/.

Rusciani L, Paradisi A, Alfano C, Chiummariello S, Rusciani A. 2006. *Cryotherapy in the treatment of keloids.* 07. http://www.ncbi.nlm.nih.gov/pubmed/16865862.

Ubel, Peter. 2014. *Is The Profit Motive Ruining American Healthcare.* 12 2. http://www.forbes.com/sites/peterubel/2014/02/12/is-the-profit-motive-ruining-american-healthcare/.

Vogt, Nancy. 2015. *African-American Media: Fact Sheet.* 04 29. http://www.journalism.org/2015/04/29/african-american-media-fact-sheet/.

Whoriskey, Peter. 2012. *As drug industry's influence over research grows, so does the potential for bias.* 11 12. http://www.washingtonpost.com/business/economy/as-drug-industrys-influence-over-research-grows-so-does-the-potential-for-bias/2012/11/24/bb64d596-1264-11e2-be82-c3411b7680a9_story.html.